**Emergency Medicine Residency Match
Selection Criteria and Programs Requirements**

By

**Match A Doc
and
Residency Guide**

I0464577

Contents

Introduction 19

Alabama 24

  University of Alabama Medical Center
Emergency Medicine Residency Program....24

Arizona 25

  University of Arizona College of Medicine at
South Campus Emergency Medicine
Residency Program 26

  Maricopa Medical Center Emergency
Medicine Residency Program 27

  University of Arizona Emergency Medicine
Residency Program 28

Arkansas...29

University of Arkansas for Medical Sciences Emergency Medicine Residency Program....29

California 30

Los Angeles County-Harbor-UCLA Medical Center Emergency Medicine Residency Program...30

University of California (San Francisco)/San Francisco General Hospital Emergency Medicine Residency Program 31

University of California (San Diego) Emergency Medicine Residency Program....32

University of California (Davis) Health System Emergency Medicine Residency Program....33

Stanford University Hospital/Kaiser Permanente Medical Center Emergency Medicine Residency Program 34

University of California (Irvine) Emergency Medicine Residency Program 35

Alameda County Medical Center Emergency Medicine Residency Program 36

University of Southern California/LAC+USC Medical Center Emergency Medicine Residency Program 37

Loma Linda University Emergency Medicine Residency Program 38

UCLA Medical Center/Olive View Emergency Medicine Residency Program 39

University of California (San Francisco)/Fresno Emergency Medicine Residency Program 40

Kaiser Permanente Southern California Emergency Medicine Residency Program....41

Kern Medical Center Emergency Medicine Residency Program 42

Kaweah Delta Health Care District (KDHCD) Emergency Medicine Residency Program....43

Colorado...44

Denver Health Medical Center Emergency Medicine Residency Program 44

Connecticut 45

Yale-New Haven Medical Center Emergency Medicine Residency Program 45

University of Connecticut Emergency Medicine Residency Program 46

Delaware 47

Christiana Care Health Services Emergency Medicine Residency Program 48

District of Columbia 49

Georgetown University Hospital/Washington
Hospital Center Emergency Medicine
Residency Program 49

George Washington University Emergency
Medicine Residency Program 50

Florida 51

University of South Florida Morsani
Emergency Medicine Residency Program....51

Orlando Health Emergency Medicine
Residency Program 52

Florida Hospital Medical Center Emergency
Medicine Residency Program 53

University of Florida College of Medicine
Jacksonville Emergency Medicine Residency
Program..54

University of Florida Emergency Medicine
Residency Program 55

Georgia..56

Medical College of Georgia Emergency
Medicine Residency Program 56

Emory University Emergency Medicine
Residency Program 57

Illinois 58

Presence Resurrection Medical Center Emergency Medicine Residency Program....58

John H Stroger Hospital of Cook County Emergency Medicine Residency Program....59

Southern Illinois University School of Medicine Emergency Medicine Residency Program...60

University of Illinois College of Medicine at Peoria Emergency Medicine Residency Program...61

Advocate Christ Medical Center Emergency Medicine Residency Program 62

University of Illinois College of Medicine at Chicago Emergency Medicine Residency Program...63

McGaw Medical Center of Northwestern University Emergency Medicine Residency Program...64

University of Chicago Emergency Medicine Residency Program 65

Indiana 65

Indiana University School of Medicine Emergency Medicine Residency Program....66

Iowa...67

University of Iowa Hospitals and Clinics Emergency Medicine Residency Program....67

Kansas 68

University of Kansas School of Medicine Emergency Medicine Residency Program....68

Kentucky...69

University of Kentucky College of Medicine Emergency Medicine Residency Program....69

University of Louisville Emergency Medicine Residency Program 70

Louisiana 71

Louisiana State University (Shreveport) Emergency Medicine Residency Program....71

Earl K Long Medical Center/Louisiana State University (Baton Rouge) Emergency Medicine Residency Program 72

Louisiana State University Emergency Medicine Residency Program 73

Maine 74

Maine Medical Center Emergency Medicine Residency Program 74

Maryland...75

University of Maryland Emergency Medicine Residency Program 75

Johns Hopkins University Emergency Medicine Residency Program 76

Massachusetts 77

Beth Israel Deaconess Medical Center/Harvard Medical School Emergency Medicine Residency Program 77

Brigham and Women's Hospital/Massachusetts General Hospital/Harvard Medical School Emergency Medicine Residency Program 78

Baystate Medical Center/Tufts University School of Medicine Emergency Medicine Residency Program 79

Boston Medical Center Emergency Medicine Residency Program 80

University of Massachusetts Emergency Medicine Residency Program 81

Michigan..82

St John Hospital and Medical Center Emergency Medicine Residency Program....82

Western Michigan University School of Medicine Emergency Medicine Residency Program..83

University of Michigan Emergency Medicine Residency Program 84

Genesys Regional Medical Center Emergency Medicine Residency Program 85

William Beaumont Hospital Emergency Medicine Residency Program 86

Detroit Medical Center/Wayne State University (Sinai-Grace Hospital) Emergency Medicine Residency Program 87

Sparrow Hospital/Michigan State University Emergency Medicine Residency Program....88

Grand Rapids Medical Education Partners/Michigan State University Emergency Medicine Residency Program....89

Henry Ford Hospital/Wayne State University Emergency Medicine Residency Program....90

Detroit Medical Center/Wayne State University (Detroit Receiving Hospital) Emergency Medicine Residency Program....91

Central Michigan University College of Medicine Emergency Medicine Residency Program..92

Minnesota 93

    Mayo Clinic College of Medicine (Rochester)
    Emergency Medicine Residency Program....93

    HealthPartners Institute for Education and
    Research Emergency Medicine Residency
    Program...94

    Hennepin County Medical Center Emergency
    Medicine Residency Program 95

Mississippi..96

    University of Mississippi Medical Center
    Emergency Medicine Residency Program....96

Missouri 97

    St Louis University School of Medicine
    Emergency Medicine Residency Program....97

    Washington University/B-JH/SLCH Emergency
    Medicine Residency Consortium 98

    University of Missouri at Kansas City
    Emergency Medicine Residency Program....99

    University of Missouri-Columbia School of
    Medicine Program.....................................100

Nebraska 101

    University of Nebraska Medical Center
    Emergency Medicine Residency Program..101

Nevada 102

    University of Nevada School of Medicine
    Emergency Medicine Residency Program..103

New Hampshire...104

    Dartmouth-Hitchcock Medical Center
    Emergency Medicine Residency Program..104

New Jersey 105

    Rutgers New Jersey Medical School
    Emergency Medicine Residency Program..105

    Rutgers Robert Wood Johnson Medical
    School Emergency Medicine Residency
    Program..106

    Newark Beth Israel Medical Center
    Emergency Medicine Residency Program..107

    Cooper Medical School of Rowan
    University/Cooper University Hospital
    Emergency Medicine Residency Program..108

    Atlantic Health (Morristown) Emergency
    Medicine Residency Program 109

    Hackensack University Medical Center
    Emergency Medicine Residency Program..110

    New York Medical College at St Joseph's
    Regional Medical Center Emergency
    Medicine Residency Program 111

New Mexico 112

    University of New Mexico Emergency
    Medicine Residency Program 112

New York..113

    New York Hospital Medical Center of
    Queens/Cornell University Medical College
    Emergency Medicine Residency Program..113

    SUNY Health Science Center at Brooklyn
    Emergency Medicine Residency Program..114

    University at Buffalo Emergency Medicine
    Residency Program 115

    Maimonides Medical Center Emergency
    Medicine Residency Program 116

    New York Methodist Hospital Emergency
    Medicine Residency Program 117

    NSLIJHS/Hofstra North Shore-LIJ School of
    Medicine at North Shore University Hospital
    Emergency Medicine Residency Program..118

    University of Rochester Emergency Medicine
    Residency Program 119

    SUNY Upstate Medical University Emergency
    Medicine Residency Program 120

Icahn School of Medicine at Mount Sinai/St Luke's-Roosevelt Hospital Center Emergency Medicine Residency Program 121

Brooklyn Hospital Center Emergency Medicine Residency Program 122

New York University School of Medicine Emergency Medicine Residency Program..123

SUNY at Stony Brook Emergency Medicine Residency Program 124

Icahn School of Medicine at Mount Sinai Emergency Medicine Residency Program..125

Albany Medical Center Emergency Medicine Residency Program 126

New York Presbyterian Hospital Emergency Medicine Residency Program 127

Staten Island University Hospital Emergency Medicine Residency Program 128

NSLIJHS/Hofstra North Shore-LIJ School of Medicine at Long Island Jewish Medical Center Emergency Medicine Residency Program...129

Lincoln Medical and Mental Health Center Emergency Medicine Residency Program..130

New York Medical College (Metropolitan) Emergency Medicine Residency Program..131

Albert Einstein College of Medicine (Jacobi/Montefiore) Emergency Medicine Residency Program 132

Icahn School of Medicine at Mount Sinai (Beth Israel) Emergency Medicine Residency Program...133

North Carolina..134

University of North Carolina Hospitals Emergency Medicine Residency Program..134

Duke University Hospital Emergency Medicine Residency Program 135

Vidant Medical Center/East Carolina University Emergency Medicine Residency Program...136

Wake Forest University School of Medicine Emergency Medicine Residency Program..137

Carolinas Medical Center Emergency Medicine Residency Program 138

Ohio..139

Case Western Reserve University (MetroHealth) Emergency Medicine Residency Program 139

Case Western Reserve University/University Hospitals Case Medical Center Emergency Medicine Residency Program 140

University of Toledo Emergency Medicine Residency Program 141

Mercy St Vincent Medical Center/Mercy Health Partners Emergency Medicine Residency Program 142

Wright State University Emergency Medicine Residency Program 143

Ohio State University Hospital Emergency Medicine Residency Program 144

University of Cincinnati Medical Center/College of Medicine Emergency Medicine Residency Program 145

Akron General Medical Center/NEOMED Emergency Medicine Residency Program..146

Summa Health System/NEOMED Emergency Medicine Residency Program 147

Oklahoma 148

University of Oklahoma College of Medicine-Tulsa Emergency Medicine Residency Program..148

Oregon 149

Oregon Health & Science University Emergency Medicine Residency Program..149

Pennsylvania 150

Penn State Milton S Hershey Medical Center Emergency Medicine Residency Program..150

Lehigh Valley Health Network/University of South Florida College of Medicine Emergency Medicine Residency Program 151

Temple University Hospital Emergency Medicine Residency Program 152

University of Pennsylvania Emergency Medicine Residency Program 153

Albert Einstein Healthcare Network Emergency Medicine Residency Program..154

St Luke's Hospital Emergency Medicine Residency Program 155

York Hospital Emergency Medicine Residency Program.....................156

Thomas Jefferson University Emergency Medicine Residency Program 157

UPMC Medical Education Emergency Medicine Residency Program 158

Allegheny General Hospital-Western Pennsylvania Hospital Medical Education

Consortium (AGH) Emergency Medicine Residency Program 159

Drexel University College of Medicine/Hahnemann University Hospital Emergency Medicine Residency Program..160

Geisinger Health System Emergency Medicine Residency Program 161

Rhode Island...162

Brown University Emergency Medicine Residency Program 162

South Carolina..163

Medical University of South Carolina Emergency Medicine Residency Program..163

Palmetto Health/University of South Carolina School of Medicine Emergency Medicine Residency Program 164

Tennessee 165

University of Tennessee College of Medicine at Chattanooga Emergency Medicine Residency Program 165

Vanderbilt University Emergency Medicine Residency Program 166

University of Tennessee College of Medicine at Murfreesboro Emergency Medicine Residency Program 167

University of Tennessee College of Medicine at Memphis Emergency Medicine Residency Program..168

Texas 169

Baylor College of Medicine Emergency Medicine Residency Program 169

University of Texas Southwestern Medical School Emergency Medicine Residency Program..170

Texas A&M College of Medicine-Scott and White Emergency Medicine Residency Program..171

University of Texas at Houston Emergency Medicine Residency Program 172

Christus Spohn Memorial Hospital Emergency Medicine Residency Program 173

John Peter Smith Hospital (Tarrant County Hospital District) Emergency Medicine Residency Program 174

Texas Tech University Health Sciences Center Paul L Foster School of Medicine Emergency Medicine Residency Program 175

University of Texas School of Medicine at San Antonio Emergency Medicine Residency Program...176

University of Texas Southwestern Medical School (Austin) Emergency Medicine Residency Program 177

Utah..178

University of Utah Emergency Medicine Residency Program 178

Virginia 179

Virginia Commonwealth University Health System Emergency Medicine Residency Program...179

University of Virginia Emergency Medicine Residency Program 180

Carilion Clinic-Virginia Tech Carilion School of Medicine Emergency Medicine Residency Program...181

Eastern Virginia Medical School Emergency Medicine Residency Program 182

Washington 183

University of Washington Emergency Medicine Residency Program 183

West Virginia 184

West Virginia University Emergency Medicine
Residency Program 185

Wisconsin..186

University of Wisconsin Emergency Medicine
Residency Program 186

Medical College of Wisconsin Affiliated
Hospitals Emergency Medicine Residency
Program...187

Introduction

Emergency Medicine Residency Match

Selection Criteria and programs requirements

This book is the must-read book and most single important piece you buy in your battle for residency. This is the **Emergency Medicine** Residency Match Selection Criteria and Programs Requirements book that contains up-to-date information about all the programs in the United States for both AMGs and IMGs. Why this book is essential to match? It has been shown that applying to programs that you don't match their minimum criteria is just waste of money and time. It is very important that you apply to those programs that you meet their requirements and this why we decided to make your life easier by gathering the information you need in one book. The information was gathered from program directors, coordinators, chiefs, faculty and residents. It includes Programs names, Programs codes, States, Addresses, Phones, Faxes, Percentage of IMGs in the programs, Minimum USMLE Step 1 and Step 2 Score Requirements, Attempts on any step, CS requirement at time of application, USCE Requirements, Cut-Off time since graduation, Programs offering couple match and Visas Sponsored or accepted. We have more than 10 years experience in the match field and our book is the proof that will help you to get the highest number of interviews to increase your chances in the match journey.

which is/are subject to change by/at the programs at any time. Although we did our best to get the most accurate information as much as possible from the program directors, coordinators, faculty and residents, however, you understand that by reading this book you are using the information here on your own responsibility.

Alabama

University of Alabama Medical Center Emergency Medicine Residency Program

Specialty: Emergency Medicine
Program name: University of Alabama Medical Center Program
Program code: 110-01-31-165
NRMP Code: 1007110C0

Program type: University-based
State: Alabama
Address: University of Alabama Medical Center, Old Hillman Building Room 246,
            619 S 19th St, Birmingham, AL 35249-7013
Phone: (205) 934-3640
Fax: (205) 996-9590
Percentage of IMGs in the program: 0%
Minimum USMLE Step 1 Score Requirement: No limits set
Minimum USMLE Step 2 Score Requirement: No limits set
Attempts on any step: Two attempts allowed maximum on each step.
CS required at time of application: Yes including ECFMG certificate
USCE Requirement: None
Cut-Off time since graduation: No limits set
Program offers couple match: Yes
Visas Sponsored or accepted: J1 visa

Arizona

University of Arizona College of Medicine at South Campus Emergency Medicine Residency Program

Specialty: Emergency Medicine
Program name: University of Arizona College of Medicine at South Campus Program
Program code: 110-03-21-203
NRMP Code: 1371110C0
Program type: University-based
State: Arizona
Address: University of Arizona College of Medicine, Suite 2254,
           3950 S Country Club, Tucson, AZ 85714
Phone: (520) 626-5582
Fax: (520) 626-2819
Percentage of IMGs in the program: 0%
Minimum USMLE Step 1 Score Requirement: 225
Minimum USMLE Step 2 Score Requirement: 225
Attempts on any step: Must pass on first attempt on any step including CS exam
CS required at time of application: No
USCE Requirement: Yes
Cut-Off time since graduation: 5 years
Program offers couple match: Yes
Visas Sponsored or accepted: J1 visa

Maricopa Medical Center Emergency Medicine Residency Program

Specialty: Emergency Medicine
Program name: Maricopa Medical Center Program
Program code: 110-03-21-082
NRMP Code: 1898110C0
Program type: Community-based University affiliated hospital
State: Arizona
Address: Maricopa Medical Center, Department of Emergency Medicine,
           2601 E Roosevelt St, Phoenix, AZ 85008
Phone: (602) 344-5808
Fax: (602) 344-5907
Percentage of IMGs in the program: 0%
Minimum USMLE Step 1 Score Requirement: 210
Minimum USMLE Step 2 Score Requirement: 210
Attempts on any step: Must pass on first attempt on any step including CS exam
CS required at time of application: No
USCE Requirement: Yes 1-2 months
Cut-Off time since graduation: 2 years

Program offers couple match: Yes
Visas Sponsored or accepted: No visa

University of Arizona Emergency Medicine Residency Program

Specialty: Emergency Medicine
Program name: University of Arizona Program
Program code: 110-03-12-056
NRMP Code: 1015110C0
Program type: University-based
State: Arizona
Address: University of Arizona Health Sciences Center, PO Box 245057,
          1501 N Campbell Ave, Tucson, AZ 85724
Phone: (520) 626-7233
Fax: (520) 626-1633
Percentage of IMGs in the program: 10%
Minimum USMLE Step 1 Score Requirement: 220
Minimum USMLE Step 2 Score Requirement: 220
Attempts on any step: Maximum of 2 attempts allowed on each step
CS required at time of application: No
USCE Requirement: None
Cut-Off time since graduation: No limits set
Program offers couple match: Yes
Visas Sponsored or accepted: J1 visa

Arkansas

University of Arkansas for Medical Sciences Emergency Medicine Residency Program

Specialty: Emergency Medicine
Program name: University of Arkansas for Medical Sciences Program
Program code: 110-04-21-071
Program type: University-based
State: Arkansas
Address: University of Arkansas for Medical Sciences, Slot 584,
                4301 W Markham St, Little Rock, AR 72205-7199
Phone: (501) 686-5516
Fax: (501) 686-8586
Percentage of IMGs in the program: 0%
Minimum USMLE Step 1 Score Requirement: 210
Minimum USMLE Step 2 Score Requirement: 210
Attempts on any step: Must pass on first attempt including CS exam
CS required at time of application: No

USCE Requirement: Yes 1 month
Cut-Off time since graduation: 2 years
Program offers couple match: Yes
Visas Sponsored or accepted: J1 visa and H1b visa

California

Los Angeles County-Harbor-UCLA Medical Center Emergency Medicine Residency Program

Specialty: Emergency Medicine
Program name: Los Angeles County-Harbor-UCLA Medical Center Program
Program code: 110-05-12-008
State: California
Address: Los Angeles County-Harbor-UCLA Medical Center, Box 21 PO Box 2910
          1000 W Carson St, Torrance, CA 90509-2910
Phone: (310) 222-3501
Fax: (310) 782-1763
Percentage of IMGs in the program: 0%
Minimum USMLE Step 1 Score Requirement: 230
Minimum USMLE Step 2 Score Requirement:

Attempts on any step: No limits set
CS required at time of application: Yes
including ECFMG certificate and PTAL/Status
letter
USCE Requirement: Yes 2-3 months
Cut-Off time since graduation: 5 years
Program offers couple match: Yes
Visas Sponsored or accepted: J1 visa

University of California (San Francisco)/San Francisco General Hospital Emergency Medicine Residency Program

Specialty: Emergency Medicine
Program name: University of California (San Francisco)/San Francisco General Hospital Program
Program code: 110-05-13-192
NRMP Code: 1062110C0
Program type: University-based
State: California
Address: UCSF Medical Center, Rm M-24,
        505 Parnassus Ave, San Francisco, CA
94143-0203
Phone: (415) 353-1529
Fax: (415) 353-8499
Percentage of IMGs in the program: 0%
Minimum USMLE Step 1 Score Requirement:

No limits set
Minimum USMLE Step 2 Score Requirement:
No limits set
Attempts on any step: No limits set
CS required at time of application: Yes
including ECFMG certificate and PTAL/Status
letter
USCE Requirement: None
Cut-Off time since graduation: No limits set
Program offers couple match: Yes
Visas Sponsored or accepted: J1 visa

University of California (San Diego) Emergency Medicine Residency Program

Specialty: Emergency Medicine
Program name: University of California (San Diego) Program
Program code: 110-05-21-080
Program type: University-based
State: California
Address: UCSD Medical Center, Department of Emergency Medicine MC 8676,
        200 W Arbor Dr, San Diego, CA 92103-8819
Phone: (619) 543-6213
Fax: (619) 543-3115

Percentage of IMGs in the program: 0%
Minimum USMLE Step 1 Score Requirement: 220
Minimum USMLE Step 2 Score Requirement: 220
Attempts on any step: Must pass on first attempt including CS exam
CS required at time of application: Yes including ECFMG certificate and PTAL/Status letter
USCE Requirement: Yes 1 month
Cut-Off time since graduation: No limits set
Program offers couple match: Yes
Visas Sponsored or accepted: J1 visa

University of California (Davis) Health System Emergency Medicine Residency Program

Specialty: Emergency Medicine
Program name: University of California (Davis) Health System Program
Program code: 110-05-21-097
NRMP Code: 1046110C0
Program type: University-based
State: California
Address: UC Davis Medical Center, PSSB 2100, 4150 V St, Sacramento, CA 95817
Phone: (916) 734-8571
Fax: (916) 734-7950

Percentage of IMGs in the program: 0%
Minimum USMLE Step 1 Score Requirement: 215
Minimum USMLE Step 2 Score Requirement: 215
Attempts on any step: Maximum of 2 attempts
CS required at time of application: Yes including ECFMG certificate and PTAL/Status letter
USCE Requirement: None
Cut-Off time since graduation: No limits set
Program offers couple match: Yes
Visas Sponsored or accepted: J1 visa

Stanford University Hospital/Kaiser Permanente Medical Center Emergency Medicine Residency Program

Specialty: Emergency Medicine
Program name: Stanford University Hospital/Kaiser Permanente Medical Center Program
Program code: 110-05-21-098
State: California
Address: Stanford University Medical Center, Division of Emergency Medicine Rm M121,
          300 Pasteur Dr, Stanford, CA 94305
Phone: (650) 723-9215
Fax: (650) 723-0121

Percentage of IMGs in the program: 0%
Minimum USMLE Step 1 Score Requirement:
No limits set
Minimum USMLE Step 2 Score Requirement:
No limits set
Attempts on any step: Must pass on first
attempt including CS exam
CS required at time of application: Yes
including ECFMG certificate and PTAL/Status
letter
USCE Requirement: None
Cut-Off time since graduation: No limits set
Program offers couple match: Yes
Visas Sponsored or accepted: H1b visa

University of California (Irvine) Emergency Medicine Residency Program

Specialty: Emergency Medicine
Program name: University of California (Irvine)
Program
Program code: 110-05-21-078
Program type: University-based
State: California
Address: UC Irvine Medical Center, Bldg 200 Rte
128-01,
        101 The City Dr S, Orange, CA 92868-
3298
Phone: (714) 456-5922

Fax: (714) 456-3714
Percentage of IMGs in the program: 0%
Minimum USMLE Step 1 Score Requirement: 230
Minimum USMLE Step 2 Score Requirement: 230
Attempts on any step: No limits set
CS required at time of application: Yes including ECFMG certificate and PTAL/Status letter
USCE Requirement: Yes
Cut-Off time since graduation: 3 years
Program offers couple match: Yes
Visas Sponsored or accepted: No visa

Alameda County Medical Center Emergency Medicine Residency Program

Specialty: Emergency Medicine
Program name: Alameda County Medical Center Program
Program code: 110-05-12-006
State: California
Address: Alameda County Medical Center Highland Hospital,
          Department of Emergency Med #22123,
          1411 E 31st St, Oakland, CA 94602-1018

Phone: (510) 437-4896
Fax: (510) 437-8322
Percentage of IMGs in the program: 0%
Minimum USMLE Step 1 Score Requirement:
No limits set
Minimum USMLE Step 2 Score Requirement:
No limits set
Attempts on any step: None
CS required at time of application: Yes
including ECFMG certificate and PTAL/Status
letter
USCE Requirement: None
Cut-Off time since graduation: 2 years
Program offers couple match: Yes
Visas Sponsored or accepted: No visa

University of Southern California/LAC+USC Medical Center Emergency Medicine Residency Program

Specialty: Emergency Medicine
Program name: University of Southern
California/LAC+USC Medical Center Program
Program code: 110-05-12-005
NRMP Code: 1033110C0
Program type: Community-based university
affiliated hospital
State: California

Address: LAC+USC Medical Center, Room 1011 GH,

1200 N State St, Los Angeles, CA 90033

Phone: (323) 226-2828
Fax: (323) 226-8101
Percentage of IMGs in the program: 0%
Minimum USMLE Step 1 Score Requirement: No limits set
Minimum USMLE Step 2 Score Requirement: No limits set
Attempts on any step: No limits set
CS required at time of application: Yes including ECFMG certificate and PTAL/Status letter
USCE Requirement: None
Cut-Off time since graduation: No limits set
Program offers couple match: Yes
Visas Sponsored or accepted: J1 visa

Loma Linda University Emergency Medicine Residency Program

Specialty: Emergency Medicine
Program name: Loma Linda University Program
Program code: 110-05-12-068
Program type: University-based
State: California
Address: Loma Linda University Medical Center, Department of Emergency Med Rm A108,

11234 Anderson St, Loma Linda, CA 92354
Phone: (909) 558-4085
Fax: (909) 558-0121
Percentage of IMGs in the program: 0%
Minimum USMLE Step 1 Score Requirement: No limits set
Minimum USMLE Step 2 Score Requirement: No limits set
Attempts on any step: No limits set
CS required at time of application: No but PTAL/Status letter required
USCE Requirement: None
Cut-Off time since graduation: No limits set
Program offers couple match: Yes
Visas Sponsored or accepted: J1 visa

UCLA Medical Center/Olive View Emergency Medicine Residency Program

Specialty: Emergency Medicine
Program name: UCLA Medical Center/Olive View Program
Program code: 110-05-12-003
State: California
Address: Ronald Reagan UCLA Medical Center, Emergency Medicine Center Suite 300,
924 Westwood Blvd, Los Angeles, CA 90024

Phone: (310) 794-0585
Fax: (310) 794-0599
Percentage of IMGs in the program: 0%
Minimum USMLE Step 1 Score Requirement: 210
Minimum USMLE Step 2 Score Requirement: 210
Attempts on any step: Must pass on first attempt on any step including CS exam
CS required at time of application: No but PTAL/Status letter required
USCE Requirement: None
Cut-Off time since graduation: No limits set
Program offers couple match: Yes
Visas Sponsored or accepted: J1 visa and H1b visa

University of California (San Francisco)/Fresno Emergency Medicine Residency Program

Specialty: Emergency Medicine
Program name: University of California (San Francisco)/Fresno Program
Program code: 110-05-12-002
NRMP Code: 1022110C0
Program type: Community-based university affiliated hospital
State: California
Address: UCSF Fresno, Emergency Medicine

Program,
> 155 N Fresno St, Fresno, CA 93701

Phone: (559) 499-6440
Fax: (559) 499-6441
Percentage of IMGs in the program: 0%
Minimum USMLE Step 1 Score Requirement: No limits set
Minimum USMLE Step 2 Score Requirement: No limits set
Attempts on any step: No limits set
CS required at time of application: Yes including ECFMG certificate and PTAL/Status letter
USCE Requirement: None
Cut-Off time since graduation: No limits set
Program offers couple match: Yes
Visas Sponsored or accepted: J1 visa

Kaiser Permanente Southern California Emergency Medicine Residency Program

Specialty: Emergency Medicine
Program name: Kaiser Permanente Southern California Program
Program code: 110-05-00-21
State: California
Address: Kaiser Permanente Southern California, Emergency Medicine Program,
> 4647 Zion Ave, San Diego, CA 92120

Phone: (619) 528-5164
Fax: (619) 528-7965
Percentage of IMGs in the program: New program
Minimum USMLE Step 1 Score Requirement: 220
Minimum USMLE Step 2 Score Requirement: 220
Attempts on any step: No limits set
CS required at time of application: Yes as will as ECFMG certificate and PTAL/ Status letter
USCE Requirement: None
Cut-Off time since graduation: No limits set
Program offers couple match: Yes
Visas Sponsored or accepted: No visa

Kern Medical Center Emergency Medicine Residency Program

Specialty: Emergency Medicine
Program name: Kern Medical Center Program
Program code: 110-05-12-001
NRMP Code: 1921110C0
Program type: Community-based university affiliated hospital
State: California
Address: Kern Medical Center, Department of Emergency Medicine,
         1700 Mount Vernon Ave, Bakersfield, CA 93306

Phone: (661) 326-2168
Fax: (661) 326-2165
Percentage of IMGs in the program: 10%
Minimum USMLE Step 1 Score Requirement: No limits set
Minimum USMLE Step 2 Score Requirement: No limits set
Attempts on any step: Must pass on first attempt including CS exam
CS required at time of application: No but PTAL/Status letter required
USCE Requirement: None
Cut-Off time since graduation: No limits set
Program offers couple match: Yes
Visas Sponsored or accepted: No visa

Kaweah Delta Health Care District (KDHCD) Emergency Medicine Residency Program

Specialty: Emergency Medicine
Program name: Kaweah Delta Health Care District (KDHCD) Program
Program code: 110-05-00-213
State: California
Address: Kaweah Delta Health Care District, Emergency Medicine Program,
        400 W Mineral King Ave, Visalia, CA 93291
Phone: (559) 624-5218

Fax: (559) 741-4845
Percentage of IMGs in the program: 18%
Minimum USMLE Step 1 Score Requirement:
No limits set
Minimum USMLE Step 2 Score Requirement:
No limits set
Attempts on any step: Maximum of 2 attempts
on each step including CS exam
CS required at time of application: Yes
including ECFMG certificate and PTAL/Status
letter
USCE Requirement: None
Cut-Off time since graduation: 3 years
Program offers couple match: Yes
Visas Sponsored or accepted: J1 visa

Colorado

Denver Health Medical Center Emergency Medicine Residency Program

Specialty: Emergency Medicine
Program name: Denver Health Medical Center
Program
Program code: 110-07-12-009
NRMP Code: 1077110C0
Program type: Community-based

State: Colorado
Address: Denver Health Medical Center, Department of Emergency Medicine MC 0108, 777 Bannock St, Denver, CO 80204-4507
Phone: (303) 602-5183
Fax: (303) 602-5184
Percentage of IMGs in the program: 0%
Minimum USMLE Step 1 Score Requirement: No limits set
Minimum USMLE Step 2 Score Requirement: No limits set
Attempts on any step: No limits set
CS required at time of application: Yes including ECFMG certificate
USCE Requirement: None
Cut-Off time since graduation: No limits set
Program offers couple match: Yes
Visas Sponsored or accepted: No visa

Connecticut

Yale-New Haven Medical Center Emergency Medicine Residency Program

Specialty: Emergency Medicine

Program name: Yale-New Haven Medical Center Program
Program code: 110-08-21-139
NRMP Code: 1089110C0
Program type: University-based
State: Connecticut
Address: Yale-New Haven Medical Center, Department of Emergency Medicine Suite 260, 464 Congress Ave, New Haven, CT 06519-1315
Phone: (203) 785-5174
Fax: (203) 785-4580
Percentage of IMGs in the program: 8%
Minimum USMLE Step 1 Score Requirement: No limits set
Minimum USMLE Step 2 Score Requirement: No limits set
Attempts on any step: No limits set
CS required at time of application: No
USCE Requirement: None
Cut-Off time since graduation: No limits set
Program offers couple match: Yes
Visas Sponsored or accepted: J1 visa

University of Connecticut Emergency Medicine Residency Program

Specialty: Emergency Medicine

Program name: University of Connecticut Program
Program code: 110-08-21-120
NRMP Code: 1094110C0
Program type: Community-based university affiliated hospital
State: Connecticut
Address: University of Connecticut Health Center, Emergency Medicine Program MC-1930, 263 Farmington Ave, Farmington, CT 06030-1930
Phone: (860) 679-4988
Fax: (860) 679-3489
Percentage of IMGs in the program: 10%
Minimum USMLE Step 1 Score Requirement: 210
Minimum USMLE Step 2 Score Requirement: 210
Attempts on any step: Must pass on first attempt including CS exam
CS required at time of application: No
USCE Requirement: Yes 1 month in any US EM Department
Cut-Off time since graduation: 5 years
Program offers couple match: Yes
Visas Sponsored or accepted: J1 visa

Delaware

Christiana Care Health Services Emergency Medicine Residency Program

Specialty: Emergency Medicine
Program name: Christiana Care Health Services Program
Program code: 110-09-12-057
NRMP Code: 1099110C0
Program type: Community-based University affiliated hospital
State: Delaware
Address: Christiana Care Health System, Department of Emergency Med PO Box 6001,
          4755 Ogletown-Stanton Rd, Newark, DE 19718
Phone: (302) 733-4176
Fax: (302) 733-1595
Percentage of IMGs in the program: 0%
Minimum USMLE Step 1 Score Requirement: No limits set
Minimum USMLE Step 2 Score Requirement: No limits set
Attempts on any step: No limits set
CS required at time of application: No
USCE Requirement: No
Cut-Off time since graduation: No limits set
Program offers couple match: Yes
Visas Sponsored or accepted: J1 visa and H1b visa

District of Columbia

Georgetown University Hospital/Washington Hospital Center Emergency Medicine Residency Program

Specialty: Emergency Medicine
Program name: Georgetown University Hospital/Washington Hospital Center Program
Program code: 110-10-12-181
NRMP Code: 1800110C0
Program type: Community-based University affiliated hospital
State: District of Columbia
Address: GUH/Washington Hospital Center, Suite NA1177 (EB 3124),
          110 Irving St NW, Washington, DC 20010
Phone: (202) 877-8080
Fax: (202) 877-7633
Percentage of IMGs in the program: 0%
Minimum USMLE Step 1 Score Requirement: No limits set
Minimum USMLE Step 2 Score Requirement: No limits set
Attempts on any step: No limits set
CS required at time of application: No

USCE Requirement: Yes, 1 month.
Cut-Off time since graduation: No limits set
Program offers couple match: Yes
Visas Sponsored or accepted: J1 visa

George Washington University Emergency Medicine Residency Program

Specialty: Emergency Medicine
Program name: George Washington University Program
Program code: 110-10-12-011
NRMP Code: 1802110C0
Program type: University-based
State: District of Columbia
Address: George Washington University Medical Center,
    Department of Emergency Medicine Suite 450,
    2120 L St NW, Washington, DC 20037
Phone: (202) 741-2914
Fax: (202) 741-2921
Percentage of IMGs in the program: 15%
Minimum USMLE Step 1 Score Requirement: No limits set
Minimum USMLE Step 2 Score Requirement: No limits set
Attempts on any step: Two maximum attempts on each step

CS required at time of application: Yes
including ECFMG certificate
USCE Requirement: Yes
Cut-Off time since graduation: No limits set
Program offers couple match: Yes
Visas Sponsored or accepted: J1 visa

Florida

University of South Florida Morsani Emergency Medicine Residency Program

Specialty: Emergency Medicine
Program name: University of South Florida
Morsani Program
Program code: 110-11-21-167
State: Florida
Address: University of South Florida, Suite 504,
One Davis Blvd, Tampa, FL 33606
Phone: (813) 627-5931
Fax: (813) 254-6440
Percentage of IMGs in the program: 10%
Minimum USMLE Step 1 Score Requirement:
No limits set
Minimum USMLE Step 2 Score Requirement:
No limits set
Attempts on any step: No limits set
CS required at time of application: No

USCE Requirement: None
Cut-Off time since graduation: No limits set
Program offers couple match: Yes
Visas Sponsored or accepted: J1 visa

Orlando Health Emergency Medicine Residency Program

Specialty: Emergency Medicine
Program name: Orlando Health Program
Program code: 110-11-21-072
NRMP Code: 1107110C0
Program type: Community-based university affiliated hospital
State: Florida
Address: Orlando Regional Medical Center,
          Department of Emergency Medicine Suite 200,
          86 W Underwood St, Orlando, FL 32806-2134
Phone: (407) 237-6329
Fax: (407) 649-3083
Percentage of IMGs in the program: 5%
Minimum USMLE Step 1 Score Requirement: 210
Minimum USMLE Step 2 Score Requirement: 210
Attempts on any step: Must pass on first attempt including CS exam
CS required at time of application: No

USCE Requirement: None
Cut-Off time since graduation: 3 years
Program offers couple match: Yes
Visas Sponsored or accepted: J1 visa

Florida Hospital Medical Center Emergency Medicine Residency Program

Specialty: Emergency Medicine
Program name: Florida Hospital Medical Center Program
Program code: 110-11-12-190
NRMP Code: 1102110C0
Program type: Community-based university affiliated hospital
State: Florida
Address: Florida Hospital, Emergency Medicine Program,
          7727 Lake Underhill Rd, Orlando, FL 32822
Phone: (407) 303-6413
Fax: (407) 303-6414
Percentage of IMGs in the program: 10%
Minimum USMLE Step 1 Score Requirement: No limits set
Minimum USMLE Step 2 Score Requirement: No limits set
Attempts on any step: No limits set
CS required at time of application: No

USCE Requirement: None
Cut-Off time since graduation: No limits set
Program offers couple match: Yes
Visas Sponsored or accepted: J1 visa and H1b visa

University of Florida College of Medicine Jacksonville Emergency Medicine Residency Program

Specialty: Emergency Medicine
Program name: University of Florida College of Medicine Jacksonville Program
Program code: 110-11-12-058
NRMP Code: 1101110C0
Program type: Community-based university affiliated hospital
State: Florida
Address: University of Florida College of Medicine Jacksonville,
        Department of Emergency Medicine Box C506,
        655 W 8th St, Jacksonville, FL 32209
Phone: (904) 244-3817
Fax: (902) 244-4077
Percentage of IMGs in the program: 0%
Minimum USMLE Step 1 Score Requirement: No limits set
Minimum USMLE Step 2 Score Requirement: No limits set

Attempts on any step: No limits set
CS required at time of application: No
USCE Requirement: None
Cut-Off time since graduation: None
Program offers couple match: Yes
Visas Sponsored or accepted: J1 visa

University of Florida Emergency Medicine Residency Program

Specialty: Emergency Medicine
Program name: University of Florida Program
Program code: 110-11-31-186
NRMP Code: 1824110C0
Program type: University-based
State: Florida
Address: University of Florida College of Medicine,
      Department of Emergency Medicine Rm 4270,
      1329 SW 16th St, Gainesville, FL 32610,
Phone: (352) 265-5911
Fax: (352) 265-5606
Percentage of IMGs in the program: 5%
Minimum USMLE Step 1 Score Requirement: No limits set
Minimum USMLE Step 2 Score Requirement: No limits set
Attempts on any step: No limits set

CS required at time of application: Yes
USCE Requirement: Yes
Cut-Off time since graduation: No limits set
Program offers couple match: Yes
Visas Sponsored or accepted: No visa

Georgia

Medical College of Georgia Emergency Medicine Residency Program

Specialty: Emergency Medicine
Program name: Medical College of Georgia Program
Program code: 110-12-21-090
NRMP Code: 1985110C0
Program type: University-based
State: Georgia
Address: Georgia Regents University MCG
            1120 15th St, Augusta, GA 30912-2800
Phone: (706) 721-2613
Fax: (706) 721-9081
Percentage of IMGs in the program: 5%
Minimum USMLE Step 1 Score Requirement: No limits set

Minimum USMLE Step 2 Score Requirement: No limits set
Attempts on any step: No limits set
CS required at time of application: No
USCE Requirement: None
Cut-Off time since graduation: No limits set
Program offers couple match: Yes
Visas Sponsored or accepted: J1 visa

Emory University Emergency Medicine Residency Program

Specialty: Emergency Medicine
Program name: Emory University Program
Program code: 110-12-12-012
NRMP Code: 1113110C0, 1113110C1
Program type: University-based
State: Georgia
Address: Grady Memorial Hospital
            49 Jesse Hill Jr Dr SE, Atlanta, GA 30303-3219
Phone: (404) 251-8865
Fax: (404) 688-6355
Percentage of IMGs in the program: 10%
Minimum USMLE Step 1 Score Requirement: No limits set
Minimum USMLE Step 2 Score Requirement: No limits set
Attempts on any step: Must pass from maximum the 2nd attempt on any step

including CS exam
CS required at time of application: No
USCE Requirement: None
Cut-Off time since graduation: No limits set
Program offers couple match: Yes
Visas Sponsored or accepted: H1b visa

Illinois

Presence Resurrection Medical Center Emergency Medicine Residency Program

Specialty: Emergency Medicine
Program name: Presence Resurrection Medical Center Program
Program code: 110-16-31-146
NRMP Code: 1937110C0
Program type: Community-based
State: Illinois
Address: Presence Resurrection Medical Center
        7435 W Talcott Ave, Chicago, IL
60631-3746
Phone: (773) 990-6550
Fax: (773) 594-7805
Percentage of IMGs in the program: 4%

Minimum USMLE Step 1 Score Requirement: No limits set
Minimum USMLE Step 2 Score Requirement: No limits set
Attempts on any step: No limits set
CS required at time of application: No
USCE Requirement: None
Cut-Off time since graduation: No limits set
Program offers couple match: Yes
Visas Sponsored or accepted: No visa

John H Stroger Hospital of Cook County Emergency Medicine Residency Program

Specialty: Emergency Medicine
Program name: John H Stroger Hospital of Cook County Program
Program code: 110-16-21-083
State: Illinois
Address: Stroger Hospital of Cook County
1900 W Polk St, Chicago, IL 60612
Phone: (312) 864-0062
Fax: (312) 864-9656
Percentage of IMGs in the program: 5%
Minimum USMLE Step 1 Score Requirement: No limits set
Minimum USMLE Step 2 Score Requirement: No limits set

Attempts on any step: Must pass on first attempt
CS required at time of application: No
USCE Requirement: Yes
Cut-Off time since graduation: No limits set
Program offers couple match: Yes
Visas Sponsored or accepted: J1 visa and H1b visa

Southern Illinois University School of Medicine Emergency Medicine Residency Program

Specialty: Emergency Medicine
Program name: Southern Illinois University School of Medicine Program
Program code: 110-16-13-204
State: Illinois
Address: Southern Illinois University School of Medicine
            701 N First St, Springfield, IL 62794-9638
Phone: (217) 545-3518
Fax: (217) 545-2711
Percentage of IMGs in the program: 0%
Minimum USMLE Step 1 Score Requirement: No limits set
Minimum USMLE Step 2 Score Requirement: No limits set
Attempts on any step: No limits set

CS required at time of application: No
USCE Requirement: None
Cut-Off time since graduation: No limits set
Program offers couple match: Yes
Visas Sponsored or accepted: J1 visa

University of Illinois College of Medicine at Peoria Emergency Medicine Residency Program

Specialty: Emergency Medicine
Program name: University of Illinois College of Medicine at Peoria Program
Program code: 110-16-12-069
NRMP Code: 1175110C0
Program type: Community-based university affiliated hospital
State: Illinois
Address: OSF St Francis Medical Center
530 NE Glen Oak Ave, Peoria, IL 61637
Phone: (309) 655-6710
Fax: (309) 624-9887
Percentage of IMGs in the program: 0%
Minimum USMLE Step 1 Score Requirement: No limits set
Minimum USMLE Step 2 Score Requirement: No limits set
Attempts on any step: No limits set
CS required at time of application: No
USCE Requirement: None

Cut-Off time since graduation: 5 years
Program offers couple match: Yes
Visas Sponsored or accepted: J1 visa

Advocate Christ Medical Center Emergency Medicine Residency Program

Specialty: Emergency Medicine
Program name: Advocate Christ Medical Center Program
Program code: 110-16-12-017
NRMP Code: 1131110C0
Program type: Community-based university affiliated hospital
State: Illinois
Address: Advocate Christ Medical Center
4440 W 95th St, Oak Lawn, IL 60453
Phone: (708) 684-5375
Fax: (708) 684-1028
Percentage of IMGs in the program: 0%
Minimum USMLE Step 1 Score Requirement: No limits set
Minimum USMLE Step 2 Score Requirement: No limits set
Attempts on any step: Must pass from first attempt including CS exam
CS required at time of application: Yes
USCE Requirement: None
Cut-Off time since graduation: 5 years

Program offers couple match: Yes
Visas Sponsored or accepted: J1 visa

University of Illinois College of Medicine at Chicago Emergency Medicine Residency Program

Specialty: Emergency Medicine
Program name: University of Illinois College of Medicine at Chicago Program
Program code: 110-16-12-016
NRMP Code: 1150110C0
Program type: University-based
State: Illinois
Address: University of Illinois Medical Center
            808 S Wood St, Chicago, IL 60612
Phone: (312) 413-7492
Fax: (312) 413-0289
Percentage of IMGs in the program: 0%
Minimum USMLE Step 1 Score Requirement: 220
Minimum USMLE Step 2 Score Requirement: 230
Attempts on any step: No limits set
CS required at time of application: Yes
USCE Requirement: Yes
Cut-Off time since graduation: 2 years
Program offers couple match: Yes
Visas Sponsored or accepted: No visa

McGaw Medical Center of Northwestern University Emergency Medicine Residency Program

Specialty: Emergency Medicine
Program name: McGaw Medical Center of Northwestern University Program
Program code: 110-16-12-015
State: Illinois
Address: Northwestern University Feinberg School of Medicine
       211 E Ontario St, Chicago, IL 60611
Phone: (312) 926-9512
Fax: (312) 926-6274
Percentage of IMGs in the program: 0%
Minimum USMLE Step 1 Score Requirement: No limits set
Minimum USMLE Step 2 Score Requirement: No limits set
Attempts on any step: No limits set
CS required at time of application: Yes including ECFMG certificate
USCE Requirement: None
Cut-Off time since graduation: No limits set
Program offers couple match: Yes
Visas Sponsored or accepted: J1 visa and H1b visa

University of Chicago Emergency Medicine Residency Program

Specialty: Emergency Medicine
Program name: University of Chicago Program
Program code: 110-16-12-014
NRMP Code: 1160110C0
Program type: University-based
State: Illinois
Address: University of Chicago Medical Center
5841 S Maryland Ave, Chicago, IL 60637
Phone: (773) 702-9109
Fax: (773) 702-3135
Percentage of IMGs in the program: 0%
Minimum USMLE Step 1 Score Requirement: No limits set
Minimum USMLE Step 2 Score Requirement: No limits set
Attempts on any step: No limits set
CS required at time of application: No
USCE Requirement: Yes, 1 month
Cut-Off time since graduation: No limits set
Program offers couple match: Yes
Visas Sponsored or accepted: J1 visa and H1b visa

Indiana

Indiana University School of Medicine Emergency Medicine Residency Program

Specialty: Emergency Medicine
Program name: Indiana University School of Medicine Program
Program code: 110-17-12-018
NRMP Code: 1187110C0
Program type: University-based
State: Indiana
Address: IU Health Methodist Hospital
          1701 N Senate Blvd, Indianapolis, IN 46202
Phone: (317) 962-5975
Fax: (317) 963-5394
Percentage of IMGs in the program: 0%
Minimum USMLE Step 1 Score Requirement: No limits set
Minimum USMLE Step 2 Score Requirement: No limits set
Attempts on any step: No limits set
CS required at time of application: No
USCE Requirement: Yes
Cut-Off time since graduation: No limits set
Program offers couple match: Yes
Visas Sponsored or accepted: J1 visa

Iowa

University of Iowa Hospitals and Clinics Emergency Medicine Residency Program

Specialty: Emergency Medicine
Program name: University of Iowa Hospitals and Clinics Program
Program code: 110-18-12-174
State: Iowa
Address: University of Iowa Hospitals and Clinics
          200 Hawkins Dr, Iowa City, IA 52242-1009
Phone: (319) 384-6511
Fax: (319) 356-1138
Percentage of IMGs in the program: 0%
Minimum USMLE Step 1 Score Requirement: No limits set
Minimum USMLE Step 2 Score Requirement: No limits set
Attempts on any step: Must pass on first attempt
CS required at time of application: Yes including ECFMG certificate
USCE Requirement: None
Cut-Off time since graduation: 10 years
Program offers couple match: Yes
Visas Sponsored or accepted: No visa

Kansas

University of Kansas School of Medicine Emergency Medicine Residency Program

Specialty: Emergency Medicine
Program name: University of Kansas School of Medicine Program
Program code: 110-19-13-182

State: Kansas
Address: University of Kansas Hospital
          3901 Rainbow Blvd, Kansas City, KS 66106
Phone: (913) 588-1559
Fax: (913) 588-9104
Percentage of IMGs in the program: 0%
Minimum USMLE Step 1 Score Requirement: No limits set
Minimum USMLE Step 2 Score Requirement: No limits set
Attempts on any step: No limits set
CS required at time of application: Yes including ECFMG certificate
USCE Requirement: None

Cut-Off time since graduation: No limits set
Program offers couple match: Yes
Visas Sponsored or accepted: J1 visa and H1b visa

Kentucky

University of Kentucky College of Medicine Emergency Medicine Residency Program

Specialty: Emergency Medicine
Program name: University of Kentucky College of Medicine Program
Program code: 110-20-21-129
State: Kentucky
Address: University of Kentucky Medical Center
800 Rose St, Lexington, KY 40536-0298
Phone: (859) 323-5083
Fax: (859) 323-8056
Percentage of IMGs in the program: 0%
Minimum USMLE Step 1 Score
Requirement: No limits set
Minimum USMLE Step 2 Score

Requirement: No limits set
Attempts on any step: No limits set
CS required at time of application: Yes
including ECFMG certificate
USCE Requirement: None
Cut-Off time since graduation: 10 years
Program offers couple match: Yes
Visas Sponsored or accepted: J1 visa

University of Louisville Emergency Medicine Residency Program

Specialty: Emergency Medicine
Program name: University of Louisville Program
Program code: 110-20-12-020
NRMP Code: 1217110C0
Program type: University-based
State: Kentucky
Address: University of Louisville Hospital
530 S Jackson St, Louisville, KY 40202
Phone: (502) 852-1273
Fax: (502) 852-0066
Percentage of IMGs in the program: 0%
Minimum USMLE Step 1 Score
Requirement: No limits set
Minimum USMLE Step 2 Score
Requirement: No limits set
Attempts on any step: No limits set
CS required at time of application: No
USCE Requirement: None

Cut-Off time since graduation: No limits set
Program offers couple match: Yes
Visas Sponsored or accepted: J1 visa

Louisiana

Louisiana State University (Shreveport) Emergency Medicine Residency Program

Specialty: Emergency Medicine
Program name: Louisiana State University (Shreveport) Program
Program code: 110-21-22-170
State: Louisiana
Address: LSU Health Science Center Shreveport
1541 Kings Highway, Shreveport, LA 71130-3932
Phone: (318) 675-6632
Fax: (318) 675-6878
Percentage of IMGs in the program: 20%
Minimum USMLE Step 1 Score Requirement: 220
Minimum USMLE Step 2 Score Requirement: 220
Attempts on any step: Must pass on maximum 2nd attempt on each step including CS exam

CS required at time of application: No
USCE Requirement: None
Cut-Off time since graduation: No limits set
Program offers couple match: Yes
Visas Sponsored or accepted: J1 visa

Earl K Long Medical Center/Louisiana State University (Baton Rouge) Emergency Medicine Residency Program

Specialty: Emergency Medicine
Program name: Earl K Long Medical Center/Louisiana State University (Baton Rouge) Program
Program code: 110-21-21-117
State: Louisiana
Address: LSU Baton Rouge
7556 Hennessy Blvd, Baton Rouge, LA 70808
Phone: (225) 374-0046
Fax: (225) 765-0961
Percentage of IMGs in the program: 15%
Minimum USMLE Step 1 Score Requirement: No limits set
Minimum USMLE Step 2 Score Requirement: No limits set
Attempts on any step: Must pass on maximum 2nd attempt on each step including CS exam
CS required at time of application: Yes

including ECFMG certificate
USCE Requirement: None
Cut-Off time since graduation: No limits set
Program offers couple match: Yes
Visas Sponsored or accepted: J1 visa

Louisiana State University Emergency Medicine Residency Program

Specialty: Emergency Medicine
Program name: Louisiana State University Program
Program code: 110-21-12-021
State: Louisiana
Address: LSU Health Science Center New Orleans
        1542 Tulane Ave, New Orleans, LA 70112
Phone: (504) 903-3594
Fax: (504) 903-4569
Percentage of IMGs in the program: 0%
Minimum USMLE Step 1 Score Requirement: No limits set
Minimum USMLE Step 2 Score Requirement: No limits set
Attempts on any step: No limits set
CS required at time of application: No
USCE Requirement: None
Cut-Off time since graduation: 5 years

Program offers couple match: Yes
Visas Sponsored or accepted: J1 visa

Maine

Maine Medical Center Emergency Medicine Residency Program

Specialty: Emergency Medicine
Program name: Maine Medical Center Program
Program code: 110-22-21-142
NRMP Code: 1236110C0
Program type: Community-based university affiliated hospital
State: Maine
Address: Maine Medical Center
          22 Bramhall St, Portland, ME 04102
Phone: (207) 662-7050
Fax: (207) 662-7054
Percentage of IMGs in the program: 0%
Minimum USMLE Step 1 Score Requirement: No limits set
Minimum USMLE Step 2 Score Requirement: No limits set
Attempts on any step: No limits set
CS required at time of application: No
USCE Requirement: None

Cut-Off time since graduation: No limits set
Program offers couple match: Yes
Visas Sponsored or accepted: J1 visa and H1b visa

Maryland

University of Maryland Emergency Medicine Residency Program

Specialty: Emergency Medicine
Program name: University of Maryland Program
Program code: 110-23-21-101
NRMP Code: 1252110C0
Program type: University-based
State: Maryland
Address: University of Maryland Medical System
        110 S Paca St, Baltimore, MD 21201
Phone: (410) 328-9702
Fax: (410) 328-8028
Percentage of IMGs in the program: 10%
Minimum USMLE Step 1 Score Requirement: No limits set
Minimum USMLE Step 2 Score Requirement: No limits set
Attempts on any step: No limits set

CS required at time of application: Yes
including ECFMG certificate
USCE Requirement: None, but preference given
to those who did Transitional/Prelim year
Cut-Off time since graduation: No limits set
Program offers couple match: Yes
Visas Sponsored or accepted: No visa

Johns Hopkins University Emergency Medicine Residency Program

Specialty: Emergency Medicine
Program name: Johns Hopkins University
Program
Program code: 110-23-12-022
State: Maryland
Address: Johns Hopkins University Hospital
1830 E Monument St, Baltimore, MD
21287-2080
Phone: (410) 955-5107
Fax: (410) 502-5146
Percentage of IMGs in the program: 0%
(Occasionally one)
Minimum USMLE Step 1 Score Requirement:
No limits set
Minimum USMLE Step 2 Score Requirement:
No limits set
Attempts on any step: Must pass on first
attempt including CS exam

CS required at time of application: Yes
including ECFMG certificate
USCE Requirement: Yes, 1 year
Cut-Off time since graduation: 2 years
Program offers couple match: Yes
Visas Sponsored or accepted: J1 visa

Massachusetts

Beth Israel Deaconess Medical Center/Harvard Medical School Emergency Medicine Residency Program

Specialty: Emergency Medicine
Program name: Beth Israel Deaconess Medical Center/Harvard Medical School Program
Program code: 110-24-31-163
NRMP Code: 1256110C0
Program type: University-based
State: Massachusetts
Address: Beth Israel Deaconess Medical Center
One Deaconess Rd, Boston, MA 02215
Phone: (617) 754-2339
Fax: (617) 754-2350
Percentage of IMGs in the program: 0%

**Minimum USMLE Step 1 Score
Requirement:** No limits set
**Minimum USMLE Step 2 Score
Requirement:** No limits set
Attempts on any step: No limits set
CS required at time of application: Yes
including ECFMG certificate
USCE Requirement: Yes
Cut-Off time since graduation: 4 years
Program offers couple match: Yes
Visas Sponsored or accepted: J1 visa and H1b
visa

Brigham and Women's Hospital/Massachusetts General Hospital/Harvard Medical School Emergency Medicine Residency Program

Specialty: Emergency Medicine
Program name: Brigham and Women's
Hospital/Massachusetts General
Hospital/Harvard Medical School Program
Program code: 110-24-21-150
State: Massachusetts
Address: Brigham and Women's Hospital
            75 Francis St, Boston, MA 02115
Phone: (617) 732-4892
Fax: (617) 582-6038

Percentage of IMGs in the program: 0%
Minimum USMLE Step 1 Score Requirement: No limits set
Minimum USMLE Step 2 Score Requirement: No limits set
Attempts on any step: No limits set
CS required at time of application: No
USCE Requirement: None
Cut-Off time since graduation: No limits set
Program offers couple match: Yes
Visas Sponsored or accepted: J1 visa (1st year) then J1 visa and H1b visa (during 2nd year)

Baystate Medical Center/Tufts University School of Medicine Emergency Medicine Residency Program

Specialty: Emergency Medicine
Program name: Baystate Medical Center/Tufts University School of Medicine Program
Program code: 110-24-21-116
NRMP Code: 1286110C0
Program type: Community-based university affiliated hospital
State: Massachusetts
Address: Baystate Medical Center
          759 Chestnut St, Springfield, MA 01199
Phone: (413) 794-5999

Fax: (413) 794-8070
Percentage of IMGs in the program: 15%
Minimum USMLE Step 1 Score Requirement: No limits set
Minimum USMLE Step 2 Score Requirement: No limits set
Attempts on any step: Must pass from maximum the 2nd attempt on each step
CS required at time of application: No
USCE Requirement: None
Cut-Off time since graduation: No limits set
Program offers couple match: Yes
Visas Sponsored or accepted: J1 visa

Boston Medical Center Emergency Medicine Residency Program

Specialty: Emergency Medicine
Program name: Boston Medical Center Program
Program code: 110-24-21-084
NRMP Code: 1257110C0
Program type: University-based
State: Massachusetts
Address: Boston University Medical Center
One Boston Medical Center Pl, Boston, MA 02118
Phone: (617) 414-4929
Fax: (617) 414-7759
Percentage of IMGs in the program: 5%

Minimum USMLE Step 1 Score Requirement: No limits set
Minimum USMLE Step 2 Score Requirement: No limits set
Attempts on any step: No limits set
CS required at time of application: Yes including ECFMG certificate
USCE Requirement: None
Cut-Off time since graduation: No limits set
Program offers couple match: Yes
Visas Sponsored or accepted: J1 visa

University of Massachusetts Emergency Medicine Residency Program

Specialty: Emergency Medicine
Program name: University of Massachusetts Program
Program code: 110-24-21-074
NRMP Code: 3050110C0
Program type: University-based
State: Massachusetts
Address: University of Massachusetts Medical School
　　　55 Lake Ave N, Worcester, MA 01655
Phone: (508) 421-1439
Fax: (508) 421-1490
Percentage of IMGs in the program: 5% variable

Minimum USMLE Step 1 Score Requirement: 210
Minimum USMLE Step 2 Score Requirement: 210
Attempts on any step: No limits set
CS required at time of application: No
USCE Requirement: None
Cut-Off time since graduation: No limits set
Program offers couple match: Yes
Visas Sponsored or accepted: J1 visa

Michigan

St John Hospital and Medical Center Emergency Medicine Residency Program

Specialty: Emergency Medicine
Program name: St John Hospital and Medical Center Program
Program code: 110-25-21-132
NRMP Code: 1915110C0
Program type: Community-based university affiliated hospital
State: Michigan
Address: St John Hospital and Medical Center 19251 Mack Ave, Grosse Pointe Woods, MI 48236
Phone: (313) 343-3875

Fax: (313) 343-7840
Percentage of IMGs in the program: 5%
Minimum USMLE Step 1 Score Requirement:
No limits set
Minimum USMLE Step 2 Score Requirement:
No limits set
Attempts on any step: Must pass on first attempt
CS required at time of application: No
USCE Requirement: None
Cut-Off time since graduation: 3 years
Program offers couple match: Yes
Visas Sponsored or accepted: J1 visa and H1b visa

Western Michigan University School of Medicine Emergency Medicine Residency Program

Specialty: Emergency Medicine
Program name: Western Michigan University School of Medicine Program
Program code: 110-25-21-124
NRMP Code: 1314110C0
Program type: Community-based University affiliated hospital
State: Michigan
Address: Western Michigan University School of Medicine
1000 Oakland Dr, Kalamazoo, MI

49008-8060
Phone: (269) 337-6600
Fax: (269) 337-6475
Percentage of IMGs in the program: 5%
Minimum USMLE Step 1 Score Requirement: No limits set
Minimum USMLE Step 2 Score Requirement: No limits set
Attempts on any step: Must pass on first attempt
CS required at time of application: No
USCE Requirement: None
Cut-Off time since graduation: 5 years
Program offers couple match: Yes
Visas Sponsored or accepted: No visa

University of Michigan Emergency Medicine Residency Program

Specialty: Emergency Medicine
Program name: University of Michigan Program
Program code: 110-25-21-106
State: Michigan
Address: University of Michigan Health System
1500 E Medical Center Dr, Ann Arbor, MI 48109-5305
Phone: (734) 763-7919
Fax: (734) 763-9298
Percentage of IMGs in the program: 0%

Minimum USMLE Step 1 Score Requirement: No limits set
Minimum USMLE Step 2 Score Requirement: No limits set
Attempts on any step: Must pass on first attempt
CS required at time of application: No
USCE Requirement: Yes, 12 months
Cut-Off time since graduation: No limits set
Program offers couple match: Yes
Visas Sponsored or accepted: J1 visa

Genesys Regional Medical Center Emergency Medicine Residency Program

Specialty: Emergency Medicine
Program name: Genesys Regional Medical Center Program
Program code: 110-25-13-196
State: Michigan
Address: Genesys Regional Medical Center
One Genesys Pkwy, Grand Blanc, MI 48439
Phone: (810) 606-6372
Fax: (810) 606-5990
Percentage of IMGs in the program: 20%
Minimum USMLE Step 1 Score Requirement: 215

Minimum USMLE Step 2 Score Requirement: 215
Attempts on any step: Must pass on first attempt on any step including CS exam
CS required at time of application: No
USCE Requirement: None
Cut-Off time since graduation: 3 years
Program offers couple match: Yes
Visas Sponsored or accepted: No visa

William Beaumont Hospital Emergency Medicine Residency Program

Specialty: Emergency Medicine
Program name: William Beaumont Hospital Program
Program code: 110-25-12-065
NRMP Code: 1978110C0
Program type: University-based
State: Michigan
Address: William Beaumont Hospital
3601 W 13 Mile Rd, Royal Oak, MI 48073
Phone: (248) 898-2001
Fax: (248) 898-2017
Percentage of IMGs in the program: 0%
Minimum USMLE Step 1 Score Requirement: No limits set

Minimum USMLE Step 2 Score Requirement: No limits set
Attempts on any step: No limits set
CS required at time of application: No but ECFMG certificate for IMGs required
USCE Requirement: Yes
Cut-Off time since graduation: No limits set
Program offers couple match: Yes
Visas Sponsored or accepted: J1 visa and H1b visa

Detroit Medical Center/Wayne State University (Sinai-Grace Hospital) Emergency Medicine Residency Program

Specialty: Emergency Medicine
Program name: Detroit Medical Center/Wayne State University (Sinai-Grace Hospital) Program
Program code: 110-25-12-059
State: Michigan
Address: Sinai-Grace Hospital
          6071 W Outer Dr, Detroit, MI 48235
Phone: (313) 966-1020
Fax: (313) 966-1024
Percentage of IMGs in the program: 0%
Minimum USMLE Step 1 Score Requirement: No limits set
Minimum USMLE Step 2 Score Requirement: No limits set

Attempts on any step: No limits set
CS required at time of application: No
USCE Requirement: None
Cut-Off time since graduation: 5 years
Program offers couple match: Yes
Visas Sponsored or accepted: J1 visa

Sparrow Hospital/Michigan State University Emergency Medicine Residency Program

Specialty: Emergency Medicine
Program name: Sparrow Hospital/Michigan State University Program
Program code: 110-25-12-027
NRMP Code: 1315110C0
Program type: Community-based university affiliated hospital
State: Michigan
Address: Sparrow Hospital
          1215 E Michigan Ave, Lansing, MI 48909
Phone: (517) 364-2583
Fax: (517) 364-3002
Percentage of IMGs in the program: 0% (occasionally one)
Minimum USMLE Step 1 Score Requirement: No limits set
Minimum USMLE Step 2 Score Requirement: No limits set

Attempts on any step: Must pass on first attempt including CS exam
CS required at time of application: Yes including ECFMG certificate
USCE Requirement: None
Cut-Off time since graduation: No limits set
Program offers couple match: Yes
Visas Sponsored or accepted: J1 visa

Grand Rapids Medical Education Partners/Michigan State University Emergency Medicine Residency Program

Specialty: Emergency Medicine
Program name: Grand Rapids Medical Education Partners/Michigan State University Program
Program code: 110-25-12-026
NRMP Code: 2077110C0
Program type: Community-based university affiliated hospital
State: Michigan
Address: Grand Rapids Med Education Partners
             100 Michigan St NE, Grand Rapids, MI 49503
Phone: (616) 391-3106
Fax: (616) 391-3674
Percentage of IMGs in the program: 0%

Minimum USMLE Step 1 Score Requirement: 205
Minimum USMLE Step 2 Score Requirement: 210
Attempts on any step: Must pass on first attempt especially CS exam
CS required at time of application: Yes including ECFMG certificate
USCE Requirement: Yes, 3 months
Cut-Off time since graduation: 5 years
Program offers couple match: Yes
Visas Sponsored or accepted: J1 visa

Henry Ford Hospital/Wayne State University Emergency Medicine Residency Program

Specialty: Emergency Medicine
Program name: Henry Ford Hospital/Wayne State University Program
Program code: 110-25-12-025
NRMP Code: 1300110C0
Program type: Community-based university affiliated hospital
State: Michigan
Address: Henry Ford Hospital
    2799 W Grand Blvd, Detroit, MI 48202
Phone: (313) 916-1553
Fax: (313) 916-7437
Percentage of IMGs in the program: 8%

Minimum USMLE Step 1 Score Requirement:
No limits set
Minimum USMLE Step 2 Score Requirement:
No limits set
Attempts on any step: No limits set
CS required at time of application: Yes
USCE Requirement: None
Cut-Off time since graduation: No limits set
Program offers couple match: Yes
Visas Sponsored or accepted: J1 visa

Detroit Medical Center/Wayne State University (Detroit Receiving Hospital) Emergency Medicine Residency Program

Specialty: Emergency Medicine
Program name: Detroit Medical Center/Wayne State University (Detroit Receiving Hospital) Program
Program code: 110-25-12-024
State: Michigan
Address: Detroit Med Ctr/Wayne State University
            4201 St Antoine Blvd, Detroit, MI 48201
Phone: (313) 993-2530
Fax: (313) 993-7703
Percentage of IMGs in the program: 0%

Minimum USMLE Step 1 Score Requirement: No limits set
Minimum USMLE Step 2 Score Requirement: No limits set
Attempts on any step: No limits set
CS required at time of application: No
USCE Requirement: Yes, 1 year
Cut-Off time since graduation: No limits set
Program offers couple match: Yes
Visas Sponsored or accepted: No visa

Central Michigan University College of Medicine Emergency Medicine Residency Program

Specialty: Emergency Medicine
Program name: Central Michigan University College of Medicine Program
Program code: 110-25-11-138
NRMP Code: 1320110C0, 1320110C1
Program type: Community-based university affiliated hospital
State: Michigan
Address: Central Michigan University College of Medicine
1000 Houghton Ave, Saginaw, MI 48602
Phone: (989) 583-6817

Fax: (989) 583-7436
Percentage of IMGs in the program: 20%
Minimum USMLE Step 1 Score Requirement: No limits set
Minimum USMLE Step 2 Score Requirement: No limits set
Attempts on any step: Must pass on first attempt on any step
CS required at time of application: No
USCE Requirement: Yes, 3 months
Cut-Off time since graduation: 2 years
Program offers couple match: Yes
Visas Sponsored or accepted: No visa

Minnesota

Mayo Clinic College of Medicine (Rochester) Emergency Medicine Residency Program

Specialty: Emergency Medicine
Program name: Mayo Clinic College of Medicine (Rochester) Program
Program code: 110-26-21-161
NRMP Code: 1328110C0
Program type: University-based
State: Minnesota

Address: St Marys Hospital
1216 Second St SW, Rochester, MN 55902
Phone: (507) 255-2192
Fax: (507) 255-6592
Percentage of IMGs in the program: 5%
Minimum USMLE Step 1 Score Requirement: No limits set
Minimum USMLE Step 2 Score Requirement: No limits set
Attempts on any step: No limits set
CS required at time of application: Yes including ECFMG certificate
USCE Requirement: None
Cut-Off time since graduation: No limits set
Program offers couple match: Yes
Visas Sponsored or accepted: J1 visa

HealthPartners Institute for Education and Research Emergency Medicine Residency Program

Specialty: Emergency Medicine
Program name: HealthPartners Institute for Education and Research Program
Program code: 110-26-21-144
NRMP Code: 1335110C0
Program type: Community-based university affiliated hospital
State: Minnesota

Address: Regions Hospital
          640 Jackson St, St Paul, MN 55101-2595
Phone: (651) 254-5091
Fax: (651) 254-5216
Percentage of IMGs in the program: 0%
Minimum USMLE Step 1 Score Requirement: No limits set
Minimum USMLE Step 2 Score Requirement: No limits set
Attempts on any step: No limits set
CS required at time of application: No
USCE Requirement: None
Cut-Off time since graduation: 5 years
Program offers couple match: Yes
Visas Sponsored or accepted: J1 visa and H1b visa

Hennepin County Medical Center Emergency Medicine Residency Program

Specialty: Emergency Medicine
Program name: Hennepin County Medical Center Program
Program code: 110-26-12-028
State: Minnesota
Address: Hennepin County Medical Center
          701 Park Ave S, Minneapolis, MN 55415

Phone: (612) 873-5645
Fax: (612) 904-4241
Percentage of IMGs in the program: 0%
Minimum USMLE Step 1 Score Requirement:
No limits set
Minimum USMLE Step 2 Score Requirement:
No limits set
Attempts on any step: No limits set
CS required at time of application: Yes
USCE Requirement: None
Cut-Off time since graduation: No limits set
Program offers couple match: Yes
Visas Sponsored or accepted: No visa

Mississippi

University of Mississippi Medical Center Emergency Medicine Residency Program

Specialty: Emergency Medicine
Program name: University of Mississippi Medical Center Program
Program code: 110-27-21-073
NRMP Code: 1957110C0
Program type: University-based
State: Mississippi

Address: University of Mississippi Med Center, Department of Emergency Medicine,
          2500 N State St, Jackson, MS 39216-4505
Phone: (601) 984-5582
Fax: (601) 984-5583
Percentage of IMGs in the program: 18%
Minimum USMLE Step 1 Score Requirement: No limits set
Minimum USMLE Step 2 Score Requirement: No limits set
Attempts on any step: Must pass on first attempt including CS exam
CS required at time of application: No
USCE Requirement: None
Cut-Off time since graduation: No limits set
Program offers couple match: Yes
Visas Sponsored or accepted: J1 visa

Missouri

St Louis University School of Medicine Emergency Medicine Residency Program

Specialty: Emergency Medicine
Program name: St Louis University School of Medicine Program

Program code: 110-28-31-201
NRMP Code:1365110M0
Program type: University-based
State: Missouri
Address: St Louis University School of Medicine
3635 Vista Ave, St Louis, MO 63110
Phone: (314) 268-7133
Fax: (314) 577-8516
Percentage of IMGs in the program: 0%
Minimum USMLE Step 1 Score Requirement:
No limits set
Minimum USMLE Step 2 Score Requirement:
No limits set
Attempts on any step: No limits set
CS required at time of application: Yes
including ECFMG certificate
USCE Requirement: None
Cut-Off time since graduation: No limits set
Program offers couple match: Yes
Visas Sponsored or accepted: J1 visa

Washington University/B-JH/SLCH Emergency Medicine Residency Consortium

Specialty: Emergency Medicine
Program name: Washington University/B-JH/SLCH Consortium
Program code: 110-28-21-154
State: Missouri

Address: Washington University Medical Center
660 S Euclid Ave, St Louis, MO 63110-1093
Phone: (314) 362-9177
Fax: (314) 362-0478
Percentage of IMGs in the program: 0%
Minimum USMLE Step 1 Score Requirement: 220
Minimum USMLE Step 2 Score Requirement: 220
Attempts on any step: Must pass maximum from 2nd attempt
CS required at time of application: Yes including ECFMG certificate
USCE Requirement: Yes, 1 month
Cut-Off time since graduation: 5 years
Program offers couple match: Yes
Visas Sponsored or accepted: J1 visa

University of Missouri at Kansas City Emergency Medicine Residency Program

Specialty: Emergency Medicine
Program name: University of Missouri at Kansas City Program
Program code: 110-28-12-029
NRMP Code: 1343110C0
Program type: University-based
State: Missouri

Address: Truman Medical Center
          2301 Holmes St, Kansas City, MO 64108
Phone: (816) 404-5075
Fax: (816) 404-5094
Percentage of IMGs in the program: 0%
Minimum USMLE Step 1 Score Requirement: No limits set
Minimum USMLE Step 2 Score Requirement: No limits set
Attempts on any step: No limits set
CS required at time of application: Yes including ECFMG certificate
USCE Requirement: None
Cut-Off time since graduation: No limits set
Program offers couple match: Yes
Visas Sponsored or accepted: No visa

University of Missouri-Columbia School of Medicine Program

Specialty: Emergency Medicine
Program name: University of Missouri-Columbia School of Medicine Program
Program code: 110-28-00-202
State: Missouri
Address: University of Missouri Hospitals and Clinics
          One Hospital Dr, Columbia, MO 65212
Phone: (573) 884-3233

Fax: (573) 884-5410
Percentage of IMGs in the program: 0%
Minimum USMLE Step 1 Score Requirement:
No limits set
Minimum USMLE Step 2 Score Requirement:
No limits set
Attempts on any step: Must pass on first
attempt including CS exam
CS required at time of application: Yes
including ECFMG certificate
USCE Requirement: Yes
Cut-Off time since graduation: No limits set
Program offers couple match: No
Visas Sponsored or accepted: J1 visa

Nebraska

University of Nebraska Medical Center Emergency Medicine Residency Program

Specialty: Emergency Medicine
Program name: University of Nebraska Medical
Center Program
Program code: 110-30-31-168

NRMP Code:1376110C0
Program type: University-based
State: Nebraska
Address: University of Nebraska Medical Center
        981150 Nebraska Med Center, Omaha,
NE 68198-1150
Phone: (402) 559-6802
Fax: (402) 559-9659
Percentage of IMGs in the program: 0%
Minimum USMLE Step 1 Score Requirement:
No limits set
Minimum USMLE Step 2 Score Requirement:
No limits set
Attempts on any step: No limits set
CS required at time of application: Yes
including ECFMG certificate
USCE Requirement: None
Cut-Off time since graduation: No limits set
Program offers couple match: Yes
Visas Sponsored or accepted: J1 visa

Nevada

University of Nevada School of Medicine Emergency Medicine Residency Program

Specialty: Emergency Medicine
Program name: University of Nevada School of Medicine Program
Program code: 110-31-31-189
NRMP Code: 2028110C0
Program type: University-based
State: Nevada
Address: University of Nevada School of Medicine
901 Rancho Ln, Las Vegas, NV 89106
Phone: (702) 383-7885
Fax: (702) 383-8235
Percentage of IMGs in the program: 0%
Minimum USMLE Step 1 Score Requirement: No limits set
Minimum USMLE Step 2 Score Requirement: No limits set
Attempts on any step: No limits set
CS required at time of application: No
USCE Requirement: None
Cut-Off time since graduation: No limits set
Program offers couple match: Yes
Visas Sponsored or accepted: J1 visa and H1b visa

New Hampshire

Dartmouth-Hitchcock Medical Center Emergency Medicine Residency Program

Specialty: Emergency Medicine
Program name: Dartmouth-Hitchcock Medical Center Program
Program code: 110-32-13-208
NRMP Code: 1377110C0
Program type: University-based
State: New Hampshire
Address: Dartmouth-Hitchcock Medical Center
One Medical Center Dr, Lebanon, NH 03756
Phone: (603) 650-7317
Fax: (603) 650-0715
Percentage of IMGs in the program: 0%
Minimum USMLE Step 1 Score Requirement: No limits set
Minimum USMLE Step 2 Score Requirement: No limits set
Attempts on any step: No limits set
CS required at time of application: No
USCE Requirement: None

Cut-Off time since graduation: No limits set
Program offers couple match: Yes
Visas Sponsored or accepted: J1 visa and H1b visa

New Jersey

Rutgers New Jersey Medical School Emergency Medicine Residency Program

Specialty: Emergency Medicine
Program name: Rutgers New Jersey Medical School Program
Program code: 110-33-31-177
NRMP Code: 1398110C0
Program type: University-based
State: New Jersey
Address: Rutgers New Jersey Medical School
30 Bergen St, Newark, NJ 07103
Phone: (973) 972-9261
Fax: (973) 972-9268
Percentage of IMGs in the program: 10% (Variable)
Minimum USMLE Step 1 Score Requirement: 210
Minimum USMLE Step 2 Score Requirement: 210

Attempts on any step: Must pass on first attempt including CS exam
CS required at time of application: Yes
USCE Requirement: Yes, 12 months
Cut-Off time since graduation: No limits set
Program offers couple match: No
Visas Sponsored or accepted: J1 visa

Rutgers Robert Wood Johnson Medical School Emergency Medicine Residency Program

Specialty: Emergency Medicine
Program name: Rutgers Robert Wood Johnson Medical School Program
Program code: 110-33-21-205
State: New Jersey
Address: Rutgers Robert Wood Johnson Medical School
          One Robert Wood Johnson Pl, New Brunswick, NJ 08901
Phone: (732) 235-4296
Fax: (732) 235-6434
Percentage of IMGs in the program: 20%
Minimum USMLE Step 1 Score Requirement: No limits set
Minimum USMLE Step 2 Score Requirement: No limits set
Attempts on any step: Must pass on first attempt

CS required at time of application: No
USCE Requirement: None
Cut-Off time since graduation: No limits set
Program offers couple match: Yes
Visas Sponsored or accepted: J1 visa

Newark Beth Israel Medical Center Emergency Medicine Residency Program

Specialty: Emergency Medicine
Program name: Newark Beth Israel Medical Center Program
Program code: 110-33-21-158
NRMP Code: 1397110C0
Program type: Community-based university affiliated hospital
State: New Jersey
Address: Newark Beth Israel Medical Centre
            201 Lyons Ave, Newark, NJ 07112
Phone: (973) 926-6671
Fax: (973) 282-0562
Percentage of IMGs in the program: 30%
Minimum USMLE Step 1 Score Requirement: No limits set
Minimum USMLE Step 2 Score Requirement: No limits set
Attempts on any step: Must pass on first attempt including CS exam
CS required at time of application: No

USCE Requirement: None
Cut-Off time since graduation: No limits set
Program offers couple match: No
Visas Sponsored or accepted: J1 visa

Cooper Medical School of Rowan University/Cooper University Hospital Emergency Medicine Residency Program

Specialty: Emergency Medicine
Program name: Cooper Medical School of Rowan University/Cooper University Hospital Program
Program code: 110-33-21-118
NRMP Code: 1380110C0
Program type: University-based
State: New Jersey
Address: Cooper Hospital-University Medical Center
            One Cooper Plaza, Camden, NJ 08103
Phone: (856) 342-2351
Fax: (856) 968-8272
Percentage of IMGs in the program: 0%
Minimum USMLE Step 1 Score Requirement: No limits set
Minimum USMLE Step 2 Score Requirement: No limits set
Attempts on any step: Must pass on first attempt including CS exam

CS required at time of application: Yes including ECFMG certificate
USCE Requirement: None
Cut-Off time since graduation: No limits set
Program offers couple match: Yes
Visas Sponsored or accepted: J1 visa

Atlantic Health (Morristown) Emergency Medicine Residency Program

Specialty: Emergency Medicine
Program name: Atlantic Health (Morristown) Program
Program code: 110-33-12-060
NRMP Code: 1394110C0
Program type: Community-based university affiliated hospital
State: New Jersey
Address: Morristown Medical Center
100 Madison Ave, Morristown, NJ 07962-1956
Phone: (973) 971-7926
Fax: (973) 290-7202
Percentage of IMGs in the program: 0%
Minimum USMLE Step 1 Score Requirement: No limits set
Minimum USMLE Step 2 Score Requirement: No limits set
Attempts on any step: No limits set

CS required at time of application: Yes including ECFMG certificate
USCE Requirement: None
Cut-Off time since graduation: No limits set
Program offers couple match: Yes
Visas Sponsored or accepted: J1 visa and H1b visa

Hackensack University Medical Center Emergency Medicine Residency Program

Specialty: Emergency Medicine
Program name: Hackensack University Medical Center Program
Program code: 110-33-00-213
Program type: University-based
State: New Jersey
Address: Hackensack University Medical Center
30 Prospect Ave, Hackensack, NJ 07601
Phone: (201) 996-3307
Fax: (201) 996-4239
Percentage of IMGs in the program: 25%
Minimum USMLE Step 1 Score Requirement: No limits set
Minimum USMLE Step 2 Score Requirement: No limits set
Attempts on any step: No limits set

CS required at time of application: Yes
including ECFMG certificate
USCE Requirement: None
Cut-Off time since graduation: No limits set
Program offers couple match: Yes
Visas Sponsored or accepted: J1 visa

New York Medical College at St Joseph's Regional Medical Center Emergency Medicine Residency Program

Specialty: Emergency Medicine
Program name: New York Medical College at St Joseph's Regional Medical Center Program
Program code: 110-33-00-212
State: New Jersey
Address: St Joseph's Regional Medical Center
703 Main St, Paterson, NJ 07503
Phone: (973) 754-2248
Fax: (973) 754-2516
Percentage of IMGs in the program: 25%
Minimum USMLE Step 1 Score Requirement:
No limits set
Minimum USMLE Step 2 Score Requirement:
No limits set
Attempts on any step: No limits set
CS required at time of application: Yes
including ECFMG certificate
USCE Requirement: None

Cut-Off time since graduation: No limits set
Program offers couple match: Yes
Visas Sponsored or accepted: J1 visa

New Mexico

University of New Mexico Emergency Medicine Residency Program

Specialty: Emergency Medicine
Program name: University of New Mexico Program
Program code: 110-34-21-075
NRMP Code: 1962110C0
Program type: University-based
State: New Mexico
Address: University of New Mexico Health Science Center
          1 Univ of New Mexico, Albuquerque, NM 87131-0001
Phone: (505) 272-6524
Fax: (505) 272-6503
Percentage of IMGs in the program: 10%
Minimum USMLE Step 1 Score Requirement: No limits set
Minimum USMLE Step 2 Score Requirement: No limits set

Attempts on any step: No limits set
CS required at time of application: Yes
including ECFMG certificate
USCE Requirement: None
Cut-Off time since graduation: No limits set
Program offers couple match: Yes
Visas Sponsored or accepted: J1 visa

New York

New York Hospital Medical Center of Queens/Cornell University Medical College Emergency Medicine Residency Program

Specialty: Emergency Medicine
Program name: New York Hospital Medical
Center of Queens/Cornell University Medical
College Program
Program code: 110-35-31-173
NRMP Code: 1822110C0
Program type: Community-based university
affiliated hospital
State: New York
Address: New York Hospital Queens
        56-45 Main St, Flushing, NY 11355
Phone: (718) 661-7305

Fax: (718) 661-7679
Percentage of IMGs in the program: 0%
Minimum USMLE Step 1 Score Requirement:
No limits set
Minimum USMLE Step 2 Score Requirement:
No limits set
Attempts on any step: No limits set
CS required at time of application: No
USCE Requirement: None
Cut-Off time since graduation: No limits set
Program offers couple match: Yes
Visas Sponsored or accepted: No visa

SUNY Health Science Center at Brooklyn Emergency Medicine Residency Program

Specialty: Emergency Medicine
Program name: SUNY Health Science Center at
Brooklyn Program
Program code: 110-35-31-135
State: New York
Address: SUNY Downstate Medical Center
            450 Clarkson Ave, Brooklyn, NY 11203
Phone: (718) 245-3318
Fax: (718) 245-4799
Percentage of IMGs in the program: 0%
(Occasionally 1 from Saudi affiliated
Universities)

Minimum USMLE Step 1 Score Requirement:
No limits set
Minimum USMLE Step 2 Score Requirement:
No limits set
Attempts on any step: No limits set
CS required at time of application: No
USCE Requirement: None
Cut-Off time since graduation: No limits set
Program offers couple match: Yes
Visas Sponsored or accepted: J1 visa and H1b visa

University at Buffalo Emergency Medicine Residency Program

Specialty: Emergency Medicine
Program name: University at Buffalo Program
Program code: 110-35-31-127
NRMP Code: 3099110C0
Program type: Community-based university affiliated hospital
State: New York
Address: Buffalo General Hospital
            100 High St, Buffalo, NY 14203-1154
Phone: (716) 859-1499
Fax: (716) 859-1555
Percentage of IMGs in the program: 0%
Minimum USMLE Step 1 Score Requirement:
No limits set

Minimum USMLE Step 2 Score Requirement:
No limits set
Attempts on any step: No limits set
CS required at time of application: No
USCE Requirement: Yes
Cut-Off time since graduation: No limits set
Program offers couple match: No
Visas Sponsored or accepted: No visa

Maimonides Medical Center Emergency Medicine Residency Program

Specialty: Emergency Medicine
Program name: Maimonides Medical Center Program
Program code: 110-35-21-164
NRMP Code: 1428110C0
Program type: Community-based university affiliated hospital
State: New York
Address: Maimonides Medical Center
          4802 Tenth Ave, Brooklyn, NY 11219
Phone: (718) 283-6029
Fax: (718) 635-7228
Percentage of IMGs in the program: 15%
Minimum USMLE Step 1 Score Requirement:
205
Minimum USMLE Step 2 Score Requirement:
205

Attempts on any step: Must pass on first attempt
CS required at time of application: No
USCE Requirement: Yes
Cut-Off time since graduation: 5 years
Program offers couple match: No
Visas Sponsored or accepted: J1 visa and H1b visa

New York Methodist Hospital Emergency Medicine Residency Program

Specialty: Emergency Medicine
Program name: New York Methodist Hospital Program
Program code: 110-35-21-147
NRMP Code: 1429110C0
Program type: Community-based university affiliated hospital
State: New York
Address: New York Methodist Hospital
506 Sixth St, Brooklyn, NY 11215
Phone: (718) 780-5042
Fax: (718) 780-3153
Percentage of IMGs in the program: 10%
Minimum USMLE Step 1 Score Requirement: No limits set
Minimum USMLE Step 2 Score Requirement: No limits set

Attempts on any step: No limits set
CS required at time of application: Yes
USCE Requirement: None
Cut-Off time since graduation: No limits set
Program offers couple match: No
Visas Sponsored or accepted: No visa

NSLIJHS/Hofstra North Shore-LIJ School of Medicine at North Shore University Hospital Emergency Medicine Residency Program

Specialty: Emergency Medicine
Program name: NSLIJHS/Hofstra North Shore-LIJ School of Medicine at North Shore University Hospital Program
Program code: 110-35-21-141
NRMP Code: 1700110C0
Program type: University-based
State: New York
Address: North Shore University Hospital
300 Community Dr, Manhasset, NY 11030
Phone: (516) 562-2925
Fax: (516) 562-3569
Percentage of IMGs in the program: 15%
Minimum USMLE Step 1 Score Requirement: No limits set
Minimum USMLE Step 2 Score Requirement: No limits set

Attempts on any step: No limits set
CS required at time of application: Yes
USCE Requirement: None
Cut-Off time since graduation: No limits set
Program offers couple match: No
Visas Sponsored or accepted: J1 visa and H1b visa

University of Rochester Emergency Medicine Residency Program

Specialty: Emergency Medicine
Program name: University of Rochester Program
Program code: 110-35-21-131
State: New York
Address: University of Rochester Medical Center
            601 Elmwood Ave, Rochester, NY 14642
Phone: (585) 463-2940
Fax: (585) 473-3516
Percentage of IMGs in the program: 0%
Minimum USMLE Step 1 Score Requirement: No limits set
Minimum USMLE Step 2 Score Requirement: No limits set
Attempts on any step: No limits set
CS required at time of application: No
USCE Requirement: None

Cut-Off time since graduation: No limits set
Program offers couple match: Yes
Visas Sponsored or accepted: J1 visa

SUNY Upstate Medical University Emergency Medicine Residency Program

Specialty: Emergency Medicine
Program name: SUNY Upstate Medical University Program
Program code: 110-35-21-121
NRMP Code: 1516110C0
Program type: University-based
State: New York
Address: SUNY Upstate Medical University
550 E Genesee St, Syracuse, NY 13202
Phone: (315) 464-4363
Fax: (315) 464-4854
Percentage of IMGs in the program: 20%
Minimum USMLE Step 1 Score Requirement: No limits set
Minimum USMLE Step 2 Score Requirement: No limits set
Attempts on any step: No limits set
CS required at time of application: Yes including ECFMG certificate
USCE Requirement: Yes, 1 month
Cut-Off time since graduation: No limits set
Program offers couple match: Yes

Visas Sponsored or accepted: J1 visa

Icahn School of Medicine at Mount Sinai/St Luke's-Roosevelt Hospital Center Emergency Medicine Residency Program

Specialty: Emergency Medicine
Program name: Icahn School of Medicine at Mount Sinai/St Luke's-Roosevelt Hospital Center Program
Program code: 110-35-21-109
NRMP Code: 2070110C0
Program type: Community-based University affiliated hospital
State: New York
Address: St Luke's-Roosevelt Hospital Center
1000 Tenth Ave, New York, NY 10019
Phone: (212) 523-8158
Fax: (212) 523-8000
Percentage of IMGs in the program: 0%
Minimum USMLE Step 1 Score Requirement: No limits set
Minimum USMLE Step 2 Score Requirement: No limits set
Attempts on any step: No limits set
CS required at time of application: Yes
USCE Requirement: Yes
Cut-Off time since graduation: No limits set
Program offers couple match: Yes

Visas Sponsored or accepted: J1 visa and H1b visa

Brooklyn Hospital Center Emergency Medicine Residency Program

Specialty: Emergency Medicine
Program name: Brooklyn Hospital Center Program
Program code: 110-35-21-093
NRMP Code: 1420110C0
Program type: Community-based university affiliated hospital
State: New York
Address: Brooklyn Hospital Center
121 DeKalb Ave, Brooklyn, NY 11201
Phone: (718) 250-8369
Fax: (718) 250-6528
Percentage of IMGs in the program: 20%
Minimum USMLE Step 1 Score Requirement: 210
Minimum USMLE Step 2 Score Requirement: 210
Attempts on any step: No limits set
CS required at time of application: No
USCE Requirement: None
Cut-Off time since graduation: No limits set
Program offers couple match: Yes
Visas Sponsored or accepted: J1 visa

New York University School of Medicine Emergency Medicine Residency Program

Specialty: Emergency Medicine
Program name: New York University School of Medicine Program
Program code: 110-35-21-092
NRMP Code: 2978110C0
Program type: Community-based University affiliated hospital
State: New York
Address: Bellevue Hospital Center
        462 First Ave, New York, NY 10016
Phone: (212) 562-4317
Fax: (212) 263-6826
Percentage of IMGs in the program: 0%
Minimum USMLE Step 1 Score Requirement: No limits set
Minimum USMLE Step 2 Score Requirement: No limits set
Attempts on any step: No limits set
CS required at time of application: No
USCE Requirement: None
Cut-Off time since graduation: No limits set
Program offers couple match: Yes
Visas Sponsored or accepted: J1 visa and H1b visa

SUNY at Stony Brook Emergency Medicine Residency Program

Specialty: Emergency Medicine
Program name: SUNY at Stony Brook Program
Program code: 110-35-21-091
State: New York
Address: SUNY Stony Brook University
HSC Level 4 Rm 080,
101 Nicolls Road, Stony Brook, NY 11794-8350
Phone: (631) 444-3880
Fax: (631) 444-3919
Percentage of IMGs in the program: 0%
Minimum USMLE Step 1 Score Requirement: No limits set
Minimum USMLE Step 2 Score Requirement: No limits set
Attempts on any step: Must pass on first attempt including CS exam
CS required at time of application: Yes including ECFMG certificate
USCE Requirement: None
Cut-Off time since graduation: No limits set
Program offers couple match: Yes
Visas Sponsored or accepted: J1 visa

Icahn School of Medicine at Mount Sinai Emergency Medicine Residency Program

Specialty: Emergency Medicine
Program name: Icahn School of Medicine at Mount Sinai Program
Program code: 110-35-21-087
NRMP Code: 1490110C0
Program type: University-based
State: New York
Address: Mount Sinai Medical Center
One Gustave L Levy Pl, New York, NY 10029
Phone: (212) 824-8069
Fax: (212) 731-7325
Percentage of IMGs in the program: 0%
Minimum USMLE Step 1 Score Requirement: No limits set
Minimum USMLE Step 2 Score Requirement: No limits set
Attempts on any step: Must pass on maximum 2nd attempt
CS required at time of application: No
USCE Requirement: Yes, 12 months
Cut-Off time since graduation: No limits set
Program offers couple match: Yes
Visas Sponsored or accepted: J1 visa and H1b visa

Albany Medical Center Emergency Medicine Residency Program

Specialty: Emergency Medicine
Program name: Albany Medical Center Program
Program code: 110-35-21-086
NRMP Code: 1414110C0
Program type: University-based
State: New York
Address: Albany Medical Center
47 New Scotland Ave, Albany, NY 12208-3479
Phone: (518) 262-4050
Fax: (518) 262-5362
Percentage of IMGs in the program: 0%
Minimum USMLE Step 1 Score Requirement: No limits set
Minimum USMLE Step 2 Score Requirement: No limits set
Attempts on any step: No limits set
CS required at time of application: No
USCE Requirement: None
Cut-Off time since graduation: No limits set
Program offers couple match: Yes
Visas Sponsored or accepted: J1 visa

New York Presbyterian Hospital Emergency Medicine Residency Program

Specialty: Emergency Medicine
Program name: New York Presbyterian Hospital Program
Program code: 110-35-13-169
NRMP Code: 1409110C0
Program type: University-based
State: New York
Address: New York Presbyterian Hospital-Cornell

        525 E 68th St, New York, NY 10021
Phone: (212) 746-0892
Fax: (212) 746-0887
Percentage of IMGs in the program: 0%
Minimum USMLE Step 1 Score Requirement: No limits set
Minimum USMLE Step 2 Score Requirement: No limits set
Attempts on any step: No limits set
CS required at time of application: No
USCE Requirement: None
Cut-Off time since graduation: 5 years
Program offers couple match: No
Visas Sponsored or accepted: J1 visa

Staten Island University Hospital Emergency Medicine Residency Program

Specialty: Emergency Medicine
Program name: Staten Island University Hospital Program
Program code: 110-35-12-206
NRMP Code: 1515110C0
Program type: Community-based university affiliated hospital
State: New York
Address: Staten Island University Hospital
475 Seaview Ave, Staten Island, NY 10305
Phone: (718) 226-1548
Fax: (718) 226-8447
Percentage of IMGs in the program: 0%
Minimum USMLE Step 1 Score Requirement: No limits set
Minimum USMLE Step 2 Score Requirement: No limits set
Attempts on any step: No limits set
CS required at time of application: No
USCE Requirement: None
Cut-Off time since graduation: No limits set
Program offers couple match: Yes
Visas Sponsored or accepted: J1 visa and H1b visa

NSLIJHS/Hofstra North Shore-LIJ School of Medicine at Long Island Jewish Medical Center Emergency Medicine Residency Program

Specialty: Emergency Medicine
Program name: NSLIJHS/Hofstra North Shore-LIJ School of Medicine at Long Island Jewish Medical Center Program
Program code: 110-35-12-062
NRMP Code: 1700110C1
Program type: Community-based university affiliated hospital
State: New York
Address: Long Island Jewish Medical Center
270-05 76th Ave, New Hyde Park, NY 11040
Phone: (718) 470-7873
Fax: (718) 470-9113
Percentage of IMGs in the program: 0%
Minimum USMLE Step 1 Score Requirement: 220
Minimum USMLE Step 2 Score Requirement: 220
Attempts on any step: Must pass on first attempt including CS exam
CS required at time of application: Yes including ECFMG certificate
USCE Requirement: None
Cut-Off time since graduation: 5 years

Program offers couple match: Yes
Visas Sponsored or accepted: J1 visa

Lincoln Medical and Mental Health Center Emergency Medicine Residency Program

Specialty: Emergency Medicine
Program name: Lincoln Medical and Mental Health Center Program
Program code: 110-35-12-053
NRMP Code: 1484110C0
Program type: Community-based university affiliated hospital
State: New York
Address: Lincoln Medical and Mental Health Center
    234 E 149th St, Bronx, NY 10451
Phone: (718) 579-6011
Fax: (718) 579-4822
Percentage of IMGs in the program: 40%
Minimum USMLE Step 1 Score Requirement: 215
Minimum USMLE Step 2 Score Requirement: 215
Attempts on any step: No limits set
CS required at time of application: Yes including ECFMG certificate
USCE Requirement: None
Cut-Off time since graduation: No limits set

Program offers couple match: No
Visas Sponsored or accepted: J1 visa

New York Medical College (Metropolitan) Emergency Medicine Residency Program

Specialty: Emergency Medicine
Program name: New York Medical College (Metropolitan) Program
Program code: 110-35-12-031
State: New York
Address: Metropolitan Hospital Center
          1901 First Ave, New York, NY 10029
Phone: (212) 423-6684
Fax: (212) 423-6383
Percentage of IMGs in the program: 35%
Minimum USMLE Step 1 Score Requirement: 220
Minimum USMLE Step 2 Score Requirement: 220
Attempts on any step: No limits set
CS required at time of application: Yes including ECFMG certificate
USCE Requirement: None but advantage given to those done rotation in their department
Cut-Off time since graduation: 3 years
Program offers couple match: Yes
Visas Sponsored or accepted: J1 visa and H1b visa

Albert Einstein College of Medicine (Jacobi/Montefiore) Emergency Medicine Residency Program

Specialty: Emergency Medicine
Program name: Albert Einstein College of Medicine (Jacobi/Montefiore) Program
Program code: 110-35-12-030
NRMP Code: 3172110C0
Program type: University-based
State: New York
Address: Jacobi Medical Center
1400 Pelham Pkwy S, Bronx, NY 10461
Phone: (718) 918-5820
Fax: (718) 918-7459
Percentage of IMGs in the program: 0% (occasionally one)
Minimum USMLE Step 1 Score Requirement: No limits set
Minimum USMLE Step 2 Score Requirement: No limits set
Attempts on any step: Must pass on first attempt including CS exam
CS required at time of application: No
USCE Requirement: None
Cut-Off time since graduation: 4 years
Program offers couple match: Yes

Visas Sponsored or accepted: J1 visa and H1b visa

Icahn School of Medicine at Mount Sinai (Beth Israel) Emergency Medicine Residency Program

Specialty: Emergency Medicine
Program name: Icahn School of Medicine at Mount Sinai (Beth Israel) Program
Program code: 110-35-11-149
NRMP Code: 1470110C0
Program type: Community-based university affiliated hospital
State: New York
Address: Beth Israel Medical Center
First Ave at 16th St, New York, NY 10003
Phone: (212) 420-3948
Fax: (212) 420-2954
Percentage of IMGs in the program: 0%
Minimum USMLE Step 1 Score Requirement: 210
Minimum USMLE Step 2 Score Requirement: 210
Attempts on any step: Must pass on first attempt
CS required at time of application: Yes including ECFMG certificate
USCE Requirement: Yes 3 months

Cut-Off time since graduation: 4 years
Program offers couple match: No
Visas Sponsored or accepted: J1 visa and H1b visa

North Carolina

University of North Carolina Hospitals Emergency Medicine Residency Program

Specialty: Emergency Medicine
Program name: University of North Carolina Hospitals Program
Program code: 110-36-21-130
NRMP Code: 1900110C0
Program type: University-based
State: North Carolina
Address: University of North Carolina Hospitals
170 Manning Dr, Chapel Hill, NC 27599-7594
Phone: (919) 966-6440
Fax: (919) 966-3049
Percentage of IMGs in the program: 0%
Minimum USMLE Step 1 Score Requirement: No limits set
Minimum USMLE Step 2 Score Requirement: No limits set

Attempts on any step: No limits set
CS required at time of application: Yes
including ECFMG certificate
USCE Requirement: None
Cut-Off time since graduation: No limits set
Program offers couple match: No
Visas Sponsored or accepted: J1 visa

Duke University Hospital Emergency Medicine Residency Program

Specialty: Emergency Medicine
Program name: Duke University Hospital
Program
Program code: 110-36-13-166
State: North Carolina
Address: Duke University Medical Center
          2301 Erwin Road, Duke North, Suite
2600, Durham, NC 27710
Phone: (919) 681-2274
Fax: (919) 668-6115
Percentage of IMGs in the program: 0-5%
(Variable)
Minimum USMLE Step 1 Score Requirement:
No limits set
Minimum USMLE Step 2 Score Requirement:
No limits set
Attempts on any step: No limits set

CS required at time of application: Yes
including ECFMG certificate
USCE Requirement: None
Cut-Off time since graduation: No limits set
Program offers couple match: Yes
Visas Sponsored or accepted: J1 visa

Vidant Medical Center/East Carolina University Emergency Medicine Residency Program

Specialty: Emergency Medicine
Program name: Vidant Medical Center/East
Carolina University Program
Program code: 110-36-12-063
NRMP Code: 3057110C0
Program type: University-based
State: North Carolina
Address: East Carolina University
600 Moye Blvd, Greenville, NC 27834
Phone: (252) 744-4184
Fax: (252) 744-4125
Percentage of IMGs in the program: 0%
Minimum USMLE Step 1 Score Requirement:
No limits set
Minimum USMLE Step 2 Score Requirement:
No limits set
Attempts on any step: No limits set
CS required at time of application: No
USCE Requirement: None

Cut-Off time since graduation: No limits set
Program offers couple match: Yes
Visas Sponsored or accepted: J1 visa

Wake Forest University School of Medicine Emergency Medicine Residency Program

Specialty: Emergency Medicine
Program name: Wake Forest University School of Medicine Program
Program code: 110-36-12-033
NRMP Code: 1537110C0
Program type: University-based
State: North Carolina
Address: Wake Forest Baptist Medical Center
Medical Center Blvd, Winston-Salem, NC 27157-1089
Phone: (336) 716-4625
Fax: (336) 716-5438
Percentage of IMGs in the program: 0%
Minimum USMLE Step 1 Score Requirement: No limits set
Minimum USMLE Step 2 Score Requirement: No limits set
Attempts on any step: No limits set
CS required at time of application: Yes
USCE Requirement: None
Cut-Off time since graduation: No limits set

Program offers couple match: Yes
Visas Sponsored or accepted: J1 visa

Carolinas Medical Center Emergency Medicine Residency Program

Specialty: Emergency Medicine
Program name: Carolinas Medical Center Program
Program code: 110-36-12-032
NRMP Code: 1527110C0
Program type: Community-based University affiliated hospital
State: North Carolina
Address: Carolinas Medical Center
1000 Blythe Blvd, Charlotte, NC 28232-2861
Phone: (704) 355-3658
Fax: (704) 355-7047
Percentage of IMGs in the program: 0%
Minimum USMLE Step 1 Score Requirement: 220
Minimum USMLE Step 2 Score Requirement: 220
Attempts on any step: No limits set
CS required at time of application: No
USCE Requirement: None
Cut-Off time since graduation: 2 years
Program offers couple match: Yes

Visas Sponsored or accepted: J1 visa and H1b visa

Ohio

Case Western Reserve University (MetroHealth) Emergency Medicine Residency Program

Specialty: Emergency Medicine
Program name: Case Western Reserve University (MetroHealth) Program
Program code: 110-38-21-110
NRMP Code: 1553110C0
Program type: University-based
State: Ohio
Address: MetroHealth Medical Center
2500 MetroHealth Dr, Cleveland, OH 44109-1998
Phone: (216) 778-5088
Fax: (216) 778-5349
Percentage of IMGs in the program: 0%
Minimum USMLE Step 1 Score Requirement: 220

Minimum USMLE Step 2 Score Requirement:
220
Attempts on any step: Must pass on first attempt including CS exam
CS required at time of application: No
USCE Requirement: None
Cut-Off time since graduation: No limits set
Program offers couple match: Yes
Visas Sponsored or accepted: J1 visa and H1b visa

Case Western Reserve University/University Hospitals Case Medical Center Emergency Medicine Residency Program

Specialty: Emergency Medicine
Program name: Case Western Reserve University/University Hospitals Case Medical Center Program
Program code: 110-38-13-200
NRMP Code: 1552110C0
Program type: University-based
State: Ohio
Address: University Hospitals Case Medical Center
          11100 Euclid Ave, Cleveland, OH 44106
Phone: (216) 844-3610

Fax: (216) 844-7783
Percentage of IMGs in the program: 0%
Minimum USMLE Step 1 Score Requirement:
220
Minimum USMLE Step 2 Score Requirement:
220
Attempts on any step: No limits set
CS required at time of application: Yes
USCE Requirement: Yes
Cut-Off time since graduation: No limits set
Program offers couple match: Yes
Visas Sponsored or accepted: J1 visa

University of Toledo Emergency Medicine Residency Program

Specialty: Emergency Medicine
Program name: University of Toledo Program
Program code: 110-38-12-198
NRMP Code: 1579110C0
Program type: University-based
State: Ohio
Address: University of Toledo Medical Center
            3045 Arlington Ave, Toledo, OH 43614
Phone: (419) 383-6369
Fax: (419) 383-3357
Percentage of IMGs in the program: 20%
Minimum USMLE Step 1 Score Requirement:
215

Minimum USMLE Step 2 Score Requirement: 215
Attempts on any step: No limits set
CS required at time of application: Yes including ECFMG certificate
USCE Requirement: None
Cut-Off time since graduation: 5 years
Program offers couple match: Yes
Visas Sponsored or accepted: No visa

Mercy St Vincent Medical Center/Mercy Health Partners Emergency Medicine Residency Program

Specialty: Emergency Medicine
Program name: Mercy St Vincent Medical Center/Mercy Health Partners Program
Program code: 110-38-12-040
State: Ohio
Address: Mercy St Vincent Medical Center
2213 Cherry St, Toledo, OH 43608
Phone: (419) 251-4724
Fax: (419) 251-2698
Percentage of IMGs in the program: 10%
Minimum USMLE Step 1 Score Requirement: No limits set
Minimum USMLE Step 2 Score Requirement: No limits set

Attempts on any step: Must pass on first attempt including CS exam
CS required at time of application: Yes including ECFMG certificate
USCE Requirement: Yes
Cut-Off time since graduation: 5 years
Program offers couple match: Yes
Visas Sponsored or accepted: J1 visa (and H1b visa for exceptional candidates)

Wright State University Emergency Medicine Residency Program

Specialty: Emergency Medicine
Program name: Wright State University Program
Program code: 110-38-12-039
NRMP Code: 2011110C0
Program type: Community-based
State: Ohio
Address: Wright State University
          3525 Southern Blvd, Kettering, OH 45429
Phone: (937) 395-8835
Fax: (937) 395-8387
Percentage of IMGs in the program: 0%
Minimum USMLE Step 1 Score Requirement: No limits set
Minimum USMLE Step 2 Score Requirement: No limits set

Attempts on any step: No limits set
CS required at time of application: Yes
including ECFMG certificate
USCE Requirement: None
Cut-Off time since graduation: No limits set
Program offers couple match: Yes
Visas Sponsored or accepted: No visa

Ohio State University Hospital Emergency Medicine Residency Program

Specialty: Emergency Medicine
Program name: Ohio State University Hospital Program
Program code: 110-38-12-038
NRMP Code: 1566110C0
Program type: University-based
State: Ohio
Address: Ohio State University Wexner Medical Center
376 W 10th Ave, Columbus, OH 43210-1252
Phone: (614) 293-3551
Fax: (614) 293-3124
Percentage of IMGs in the program: 0%
Minimum USMLE Step 1 Score Requirement: No limits set
Minimum USMLE Step 2 Score Requirement: No limits set

Attempts on any step: No limits set
CS required at time of application: No
USCE Requirement: None
Cut-Off time since graduation: No limits set
Program offers couple match: Yes
Visas Sponsored or accepted: J1 visa and H1b visa

University of Cincinnati Medical Center/College of Medicine Emergency Medicine Residency Program

Specialty: Emergency Medicine
Program name: University of Cincinnati Medical Center/College of Medicine Program
Program code: 110-38-12-036
NRMP Code: 1548110C0
Program type: University-based
State: Ohio
Address: University Hospital University of Cincinnati
          231 Albert Sabin Way, Cincinnati, OH 45267-0769
Phone: (513) 558-8114
Fax: (513) 558-5791
Percentage of IMGs in the program: 0%
Minimum USMLE Step 1 Score Requirement: No limits set

Minimum USMLE Step 2 Score Requirement:
No limits set
Attempts on any step: Must pass on maximum
2nd attempt
CS required at time of application: Yes
including ECFMG certificate
USCE Requirement: None
Cut-Off time since graduation: 2 years
Program offers couple match: Yes
Visas Sponsored or accepted: J1 visa

Akron General Medical Center/NEOMED Emergency Medicine Residency Program

Specialty: Emergency Medicine
Program name: Akron General Medical
Center/NEOMED Program
Program code: 110-38-12-035
State: Ohio
Address: Akron General Medical Center
        400 Wabash Ave, Akron, OH 44307
Phone: (330) 344-6326
Fax: (330) 253-8293
Percentage of IMGs in the program: 0-5%
(variable)
Minimum USMLE Step 1 Score Requirement:
220
Minimum USMLE Step 2 Score Requirement:
220

Attempts on any step: Must pass on first attempt
CS required at time of application: No
USCE Requirement: None
Cut-Off time since graduation: 5 years
Program offers couple match: Yes
Visas Sponsored or accepted: J1 visa and H1b visa

Summa Health System/NEOMED Emergency Medicine Residency Program

Specialty: Emergency Medicine
Program name: Summa Health System/NEOMED Program
Program code: 110-38-12-034
NRMP Code: 1541110C0
Program type: Community-based university affiliated hospital
State: Ohio
Address: Summa Akron City Hospital
525 E Market St, Akron, OH 44309
Phone: (330) 375-4021
Fax: (330) 375-7564
Percentage of IMGs in the program: 15%
Minimum USMLE Step 1 Score Requirement: No limits set
Minimum USMLE Step 2 Score Requirement: No limits set

Attempts on any step: No limits set
CS required at time of application: Yes
USCE Requirement: None
Cut-Off time since graduation: 4 years
Program offers couple match: Yes
Visas Sponsored or accepted: J1 visa

Oklahoma

University of Oklahoma College of Medicine-Tulsa Emergency Medicine Residency Program

Specialty: Emergency Medicine
Program name: University of Oklahoma College of Medicine-Tulsa Program
Program code: 110-39-31-193
State: Oklahoma
Address: OU School of Community Medicine
1145 S Utica Ave, Tulsa, OK 74104
Phone: (918) 579-2367
Fax: (918) 579-2369
Percentage of IMGs in the program: 0%
Minimum USMLE Step 1 Score Requirement: No limits set

Minimum USMLE Step 2 Score Requirement: No limits set
Attempts on any step: No limits set
CS required at time of application: Yes including ECFMG certificate
USCE Requirement: None
Cut-Off time since graduation: No limit set
Program offers couple match: Yes
Visas Sponsored or accepted: J1 visa

Oregon

Oregon Health & Science University Emergency Medicine Residency Program

Specialty: Emergency Medicine
Program name: Oregon Health & Science University Program
Program code: 110-40-12-042
NRMP Code: 1599110C0
Program type: University-based
State: Oregon
Address: Oregon Health & Science University
        3181 SW Sam Jackson Park Rd,
Portland, OR 97239-3098

Phone: (503) 494-7010
Fax: (503) 494-8237
Percentage of IMGs in the program: 0%
Minimum USMLE Step 1 Score Requirement:
No limits set (prefer >200)
Minimum USMLE Step 2 Score Requirement:
No limits set (prefer >210)
Attempts on any step: No limits set
CS required at time of application: No
USCE Requirement: Yes, 1 month
Cut-Off time since graduation: 5 years
Program offers couple match: Yes
Visas Sponsored or accepted: J1 visa and H1b
visa

Pennsylvania

Penn State Milton S Hershey Medical Center Emergency Medicine Residency Program

Specialty: Emergency Medicine
Program name: Penn State Milton S Hershey
Medical Center Program
Program code: 110-41-33-171
NRMP Code: 1617110C0
Program type: University-based
State: Pennsylvania

Address: Penn State Hershey Medical Center
500 University Dr, Hershey, PA 17033
Phone: (717) 531-1443
Fax: (717) 531-4441
Percentage of IMGs in the program: 10%
Minimum USMLE Step 1 Score Requirement:
No limits set
Minimum USMLE Step 2 Score Requirement:
No limits set
Attempts on any step: Must pass on first attempt
CS required at time of application: No
USCE Requirement: None
Cut-Off time since graduation: 5 years
Program offers couple match: Yes
Visas Sponsored or accepted: J1 visa

Lehigh Valley Health Network/University of South Florida College of Medicine Emergency Medicine Residency Program

Specialty: Emergency Medicine
Program name: Lehigh Valley Health Network/University of South Florida College of Medicine Program
Program code: 110-41-21-199

NRMP Code: 1601110C0
Program type: Community-based university affiliated hospital
State: Pennsylvania
Address: Lehigh Valley Hosp (Muhlenberg)
          2545 Schoenersville Rd, Bethlehem, PA 18017
Phone: (484) 884-2888
Fax: (484) 884-2885
Percentage of IMGs in the program: 5%
Minimum USMLE Step 1 Score Requirement: No limits set
Minimum USMLE Step 2 Score Requirement: No limits set
Attempts on any step: Must pass on first attempt including CS exam
CS required at time of application: Yes
USCE Requirement: None
Cut-Off time since graduation: No limits set
Program offers couple match: Yes
Visas Sponsored or accepted: J1 visa

Temple University Hospital Emergency Medicine Residency Program

Specialty: Emergency Medicine
Program name: Temple University Hospital Program
Program code: 110-41-21-155

NRMP Code: 1646110C0
Program type: University-based
State: Pennsylvania
Address: Temple University Hospital
3401 N Broad St, Philadelphia, PA 19140
Phone: (215) 707-5435
Fax: (215) 707-3494
Percentage of IMGs in the program: 0%
Minimum USMLE Step 1 Score Requirement: No limits set
Minimum USMLE Step 2 Score Requirement: No limits set
Attempts on any step: No limits set
CS required at time of application: No
USCE Requirement: None
Cut-Off time since graduation: No limits set
Program offers couple match: Yes
Visas Sponsored or accepted: J1 visa and H1b visa

University of Pennsylvania Emergency Medicine Residency Program

Specialty: Emergency Medicine
Program name: University of Pennsylvania Program
Program code: 110-41-21-148
State: Pennsylvania

Address: Hospital of University of Pennsylvania
Dept of Emergency Med Ground Ravdin
3400 Spruce St
Philadelphia, PA 19104
Phone: (215) 662-6305
Fax: (215) 662-2875
Percentage of IMGs in the program: 0%
(occasionally one)
Minimum USMLE Step 1 Score Requirement:
No limits set
Minimum USMLE Step 2 Score Requirement:
No limits set
Attempts on any step: No limits set
CS required at time of application: No
USCE Requirement: None
Cut-Off time since graduation: 4 years
Program offers couple match: Yes
Visas Sponsored or accepted: J1 visa and H1b
visa

Albert Einstein Healthcare Network Emergency Medicine Residency Program

Specialty: Emergency Medicine
Program name: Albert Einstein Healthcare
Network Program
Program code: 110-41-21-122
NRMP Code: 1631110C0
Program type: Community-based university

affiliated hospital
State: Pennsylvania
Address: Albert Einstein Medical Center
        5501 Old York Rd, Philadelphia, PA
19141
Phone: (215) 456-6336
Fax: (215) 456-6601
Percentage of IMGs in the program: 5%
Minimum USMLE Step 1 Score Requirement:
No limits set
Minimum USMLE Step 2 Score Requirement:
No limits set
Attempts on any step: No limits set
CS required at time of application: Yes
including ECFMG certificate
USCE Requirement: None
Cut-Off time since graduation: No limits set
Program offers couple match: Yes
Visas Sponsored or accepted: J1 visa and H1b
visa

St Luke's Hospital Emergency Medicine Residency Program

Specialty: Emergency Medicine
Program name: St Luke's Hospital Program
Program code: 110-41-21-111
State: Pennsylvania
Address: St Luke's University Hospital
        801 Ostrum St, Bethlehem, PA 18015

Phone: (484) 526-4903
Fax: (484) 526-2153
Percentage of IMGs in the program: 0%
Minimum USMLE Step 1 Score Requirement: No limits set
Minimum USMLE Step 2 Score Requirement: No limits set
Attempts on any step: No limits set
CS required at time of application: No
USCE Requirement: None
Cut-Off time since graduation: No limits set
Program offers couple match: Yes
Visas Sponsored or accepted: J1 visa and H1b visa

York Hospital Emergency Medicine Residency Program

Specialty: Emergency Medicine
Program name: York Hospital Program
Program code: 110-41-21-089
NRMP Code: 1674110C0
Program type: Community-based University affiliated hospital
State: Pennsylvania
Address: York Hospital
            1001 S George St, York, PA 17405
Phone: (717) 851-5064
Fax: (717) 851-3469
Percentage of IMGs in the program: 10%

Minimum USMLE Step 1 Score Requirement:
No limits set
Minimum USMLE Step 2 Score Requirement:
No limits set
Attempts on any step: No limits set
CS required at time of application: No
USCE Requirement: Yes including two SLOR
Cut-Off time since graduation: No limits set
Program offers couple match: Yes
Visas Sponsored or accepted: J1 visa and H1b visa

Thomas Jefferson University Emergency Medicine Residency Program

Specialty: Emergency Medicine
Program name: Thomas Jefferson University Program
Program code: 110-41-12-064
NRMP Code: 1630110C0
Program type: University-based
State: Pennsylvania
Address: Thomas Jefferson University Hospital
1020 Sansom St, Philadelphia, PA 19107
Phone: (215) 955-9837
Fax: (215) 955-9870
Percentage of IMGs in the program: 10%

Minimum USMLE Step 1 Score Requirement: No limits set
Minimum USMLE Step 2 Score Requirement: No limits set
Attempts on any step: No limits set
CS required at time of application: No
USCE Requirement: None
Cut-Off time since graduation: No limits set
Program offers couple match: Yes
Visas Sponsored or accepted: J1 visa and H1b visa

UPMC Medical Education Emergency Medicine Residency Program

Specialty: Emergency Medicine
Program name: UPMC Medical Education Program
Program code: 110-41-12-055
NRMP Code: 1652110C0
Program type: University-based
State: Pennsylvania
Address: University of Pittsburgh
230 McKee Pl, Pittsburgh, PA 15213
Phone: (412) 647-8284
Fax: (412) 647-8225
Percentage of IMGs in the program: 0%
Minimum USMLE Step 1 Score Requirement: No limits set

Minimum USMLE Step 2 Score Requirement:
No limits set
Attempts on any step: No limits set
CS required at time of application: No
USCE Requirement: None
Cut-Off time since graduation: No limits set
Program offers couple match: Yes
Visas Sponsored or accepted: J1 visa

Allegheny General Hospital-Western Pennsylvania Hospital Medical Education Consortium (AGH) Emergency Medicine Residency Program

Specialty: Emergency Medicine
Program name: Allegheny General Hospital-Western Pennsylvania Hospital Medical Education Consortium (AGH) Program
Program code: 110-41-12-054
NRMP Code: 1648110C0
Program type: Community-based university affiliated hospital
State: Pennsylvania
Address: Allegheny General Hospital
          320 E North Ave, Pittsburgh, PA 15212-9986
Phone: (412) 359-4905

Fax: (412) 359-4963
Percentage of IMGs in the program: 0%
Minimum USMLE Step 1 Score Requirement: No limits set
Minimum USMLE Step 2 Score Requirement: No limits set
Attempts on any step: No limits set
CS required at time of application: Yes including ECFMG certificate
USCE Requirement: None
Cut-Off time since graduation: No limits set
Program offers couple match: Yes
Visas Sponsored or accepted: J1 visa

Drexel University College of Medicine/Hahnemann University Hospital Emergency Medicine Residency Program

Specialty: Emergency Medicine
Program name: Drexel University College of Medicine/Hahnemann University Hospital Program
Program code: 110-41-12-045
NRMP Code: 1849110C0
Program type: University-based
State: Pennsylvania
Address: Hahnemann University Hospital
          245 N 15th St, Philadelphia, PA 19102
Phone: (215) 762-2365

Fax: (215) 762-1307
Percentage of IMGs in the program: 0%
Minimum USMLE Step 1 Score Requirement:
No limits set
Minimum USMLE Step 2 Score Requirement:
No limits set
Attempts on any step: Must pass on first
attempt including CS exam
CS required at time of application: No
USCE Requirement: None
Cut-Off time since graduation: No limits set
Program offers couple match: Yes
Visas Sponsored or accepted: J1 visa

Geisinger Health System Emergency Medicine Residency Program

Specialty: Emergency Medicine
Program name: Geisinger Health System
Program
Program code: 110-41-12-043
NRMP Code: 1608110C0
Program type: Community-based university
affiliated hospital
State: Pennsylvania
Address: Geisinger Health System
          100 N Academy Ave, Danville, PA
17822
Phone: (570) 271-6812

Fax: (570) 214-9442
Percentage of IMGs in the program: 0%
Minimum USMLE Step 1 Score Requirement:
No limits set
Minimum USMLE Step 2 Score Requirement:
No limits set
Attempts on any step: No limits set
CS required at time of application: No
USCE Requirement: None
Cut-Off time since graduation: No limits set
Program offers couple match: Yes
Visas Sponsored or accepted: J1 visa

Rhode Island

Brown University Emergency Medicine Residency Program

Specialty: Emergency Medicine
Program name: Brown University Program
Program code: 110-43-21-114
NRMP Code: 1677110C0
Program type: University-based
State: Rhode Island
Address: Rhode Island Hospital
         593 Eddy St, Providence, RI 02903
Phone: (401) 444-6489

Fax: (401) 444-6662
Percentage of IMGs in the program: 0%
Minimum USMLE Step 1 Score Requirement: No limits set
Minimum USMLE Step 2 Score Requirement: No limits set
Attempts on any step: No limits set
CS required at time of application: No
USCE Requirement: None
Cut-Off time since graduation: No limits set
Program offers couple match: Yes
Visas Sponsored or accepted: J1 visa and H1b for those already have it

South Carolina

Medical University of South Carolina Emergency Medicine Residency Program

Specialty: Emergency Medicine
Program name: Medical University of South Carolina Program
Program code: 110-45-12-183
NRMP Code: 1680110C0
Program type: University-based
State: South Carolina

Address: Medical University of South Carolina
169 Ashley Ave, Charleston, SC 29425
Phone: (843) 876-8023
Fax: (843) 792-9616
Percentage of IMGs in the program: 0%
Minimum USMLE Step 1 Score Requirement:
210
Minimum USMLE Step 2 Score Requirement:
210
Attempts on any step: Must pass on first
attempt
CS required at time of application: Yes
including ECFMG certificate
USCE Requirement: Yes
Cut-Off time since graduation: 5 years
Program offers couple match: Yes
Visas Sponsored or accepted: J1 visa and H1b
visa

Palmetto Health/University of South Carolina School of Medicine Emergency Medicine Residency Program

Specialty: Emergency Medicine
Program name: Palmetto Health/University of
South Carolina School of Medicine Program
Program code: 110-45-12-047
NRMP Code: 1681110C0
Program type: Community-based University

affiliated hospital
State: South Carolina
Address: Palmetto Health Richland
14 Richland Medical Park, Columbia,
SC 29203
Phone: (803) 434-3790
Fax: (803) 434-3946
Percentage of IMGs in the program: 0%
Minimum USMLE Step 1 Score Requirement:
No limits set
Minimum USMLE Step 2 Score Requirement:
No limits set
Attempts on any step: Must pass on first
attempt
CS required at time of application: Yes
USCE Requirement: Yes
Cut-Off time since graduation: No limits set
Program offers couple match: Yes
Visas Sponsored or accepted: J1 visa

Tennessee

University of Tennessee College of Medicine at Chattanooga Emergency Medicine Residency Program

Specialty: Emergency Medicine

Program name: University of Tennessee College of Medicine at Chattanooga Program
Program code: 110-47-21-195
NRMP Code: 1689110C0
Program type: Community-based university affiliated hospital
State: Tennessee
Address: Erlanger Medical Center
975 E Third St, Chattanooga, TN 37403
Phone: (423) 778-7628
Fax: (423) 778-7677
Percentage of IMGs in the program: 0%
Minimum USMLE Step 1 Score Requirement: No limits set
Minimum USMLE Step 2 Score Requirement: No limits set
Attempts on any step: No limits set
CS required at time of application: No
USCE Requirement: None
Cut-Off time since graduation: No limits set
Program offers couple match: Yes
Visas Sponsored or accepted: J1 visa and H1b visa

Vanderbilt University Emergency Medicine Residency Program

Specialty: Emergency Medicine
Program name: Vanderbilt University Program
Program code: 110-47-21-113

NRMP Code: 1702110C0
Program type: University-based
State: Tennessee
Address: Vanderbilt University Medical Center
1313 21st Ave S, Nashville, TN 37232-4700
Phone: (615) 936-1160
Fax: (615) 936-1316
Percentage of IMGs in the program: 0%
Minimum USMLE Step 1 Score Requirement: No limits set
Minimum USMLE Step 2 Score Requirement: No limits set
Attempts on any step: Must pass on first attempt
CS required at time of application: No
USCE Requirement: None
Cut-Off time since graduation: No limits set
Program offers couple match: Yes
Visas Sponsored or accepted: J1 visa

University of Tennessee College of Medicine at Murfreesboro Emergency Medicine Residency Program

Specialty: Emergency Medicine
Program name: University of Tennessee College of Medicine at Murfreesboro Program
Program code: 110-47-00-197

Program type: Community-based university affiliated hospital
State: Tennessee
Address: St Thomas-Rutherford Hospital
1840 Medical Center Pkwy,
Murfreesboro, TN 37129
Phone: (615) 396-6449
Percentage of IMGs in the program: 0% expected (still new program)
Minimum USMLE Step 1 Score Requirement: No limits set
Minimum USMLE Step 2 Score Requirement: No limits set
Attempts on any step: No limits set
CS required at time of application: Yes including ECFMG certificate
USCE Requirement: At least 1year
Cut-Off time since graduation: No limits set
Program offers couple match: Yes
Visas Sponsored or accepted: J1 visa

University of Tennessee College of Medicine at Memphis Emergency Medicine Residency Program

Specialty: Emergency Medicine
Program name: University of Tennessee College of Medicine at Memphis Program
Program code: 110-47-00-196
State: Tennessee

Address: University of Tennessee College of Medicine
　　　1265 Union Ave, Memphis, TN 38104
Phone: (423) 778-7628
Fax: (423) 778-7677
Percentage of IMGs in the program: 0% expected (still new program)
Minimum USMLE Step 1 Score Requirement: No limits set
Minimum USMLE Step 2 Score Requirement: No limits set
Attempts on any step: No limits set
CS required at time of application: No
USCE Requirement: None
Cut-Off time since graduation: No limits set
Program offers couple match: Yes
Visas Sponsored or accepted: J1 visa

Texas

Baylor College of Medicine Emergency Medicine Residency Program

Specialty: Emergency Medicine
Program name: Baylor College of Medicine Program

Program code: 110-48-21-207
State: Texas
Address: Baylor College of Medicine
1504 Taub Loop, Houston, TX 77030
Phone: (713) 873-2626
Fax: (713) 873-2325
Percentage of IMGs in the program: 10%
Minimum USMLE Step 1 Score Requirement:
No limits set
Minimum USMLE Step 2 Score Requirement:
No limits set
Attempts on any step: No limits set
CS required at time of application: No
USCE Requirement: None
Cut-Off time since graduation: No limits set
Program offers couple match: Yes
Visas Sponsored or accepted: J1 visa and H1b
visa

University of Texas Southwestern Medical School Emergency Medicine Residency Program

Specialty: Emergency Medicine
Program name: University of Texas
Southwestern Medical School Program
Program code: 110-48-21-153
NRMP Code: 2835110C0
Program type: University-based
State: Texas

Address: University of Texas Southwestern Medical Center
          5323 Harry Hines Blvd, Dallas, TX 75390-8579
Phone: (214) 648-2672
Fax: (214) 648-2683
Percentage of IMGs in the program: 0%
Minimum USMLE Step 1 Score Requirement: 215 (220 for IMGs)
Minimum USMLE Step 2 Score Requirement: 215 (220 for IMGs)
Attempts on any step: Must pass on first attempt including CS exam
CS required at time of application: Yes including ECFNG certificate
USCE Requirement: Yes, including an ER US LOR
Cut-Off time since graduation: No limits set
Program offers couple match: Yes
Visas Sponsored or accepted: J1 visa

Texas A&M College of Medicine-Scott and White Emergency Medicine Residency Program

Specialty: Emergency Medicine
Program name: Texas A&M College of Medicine-Scott and White Program
Program code: 110-48-21-102
NRMP Code: 1725110C0
Program type: Community-based university

affiliated hospital
State: Texas
Address: Scott and White Memorial Hospital
2401 S 31st St, Temple, TX 76508-0001
Phone: (254) 724-5815
Fax: (254) 724-0408
Percentage of IMGs in the program: 0%
Minimum USMLE Step 1 Score Requirement:
No limits set
Minimum USMLE Step 2 Score Requirement:
No limits set
Attempts on any step: Must pass on first
attempt
CS required at time of application: Yes
including ECFMG certificate
USCE Requirement: None
Cut-Off time since graduation: No limits set
Program offers couple match: Yes
Visas Sponsored or accepted: J1 visa

University of Texas at Houston Emergency Medicine Residency Program

Specialty: Emergency Medicine
Program name: University of Texas at Houston
Program
Program code: 110-48-21-096

NRMP Code: 2923110C0
Program type: University-based
State: Texas
Address: University of Texas HSC Houston
6431 Fannin St, Houston, TX 77030
Phone: (713) 500-5903
Fax: (713) 500-0758
Percentage of IMGs in the program: 0%
(occasionally 1)
Minimum USMLE Step 1 Score Requirement:
No limits set
Minimum USMLE Step 2 Score Requirement:
No limits set
Attempts on any step: Must pass on maximum
the 3rd attempt
CS required at time of application: Yes
including ECFMG certificate
USCE Requirement: None
Cut-Off time since graduation: No limits set
Program offers couple match: Yes
Visas Sponsored or accepted: J1 visa

Christus Spohn Memorial Hospital Emergency Medicine Residency Program

Specialty: Emergency Medicine
Program name: Christus Spohn Memorial
Hospital Program
Program code: 110-48-13-188

NRMP Code: 1705110C0
Program type: Community-based University affiliated hospital
State: Texas
Address: Christus Spohn Memorial Hospital
2606 Hospital Blvd, Corpus Christi, TX 78405
Phone: (361) 902-6762
Fax: (361) 902-4715
Percentage of IMGs in the program: 0%
Minimum USMLE Step 1 Score Requirement: No limits set
Minimum USMLE Step 2 Score Requirement: No limits set
Attempts on any step: Must pass on first attempt
CS required at time of application: Yes
USCE Requirement: Yes
Cut-Off time since graduation: 5 years
Program offers couple match: Yes
Visas Sponsored or accepted: No visa

John Peter Smith Hospital (Tarrant County Hospital District) Emergency Medicine Residency Program

Specialty: Emergency Medicine
Program name: John Peter Smith Hospital (Tarrant County Hospital District) Program

Program code: 110-48-12-202
State: Texas
Address: John Peter Smith Hospital
1500 S Main St, Fort Worth, TX 76104
Phone: (817) 702-5613
Fax: (817) 702-1143
Percentage of IMGs in the program: 10%
Minimum USMLE Step 1 Score Requirement:
No limits set
Minimum USMLE Step 2 Score Requirement:
No limits set
Attempts on any step: No limits set
CS required at time of application: Yes
including ECFMG certificate
USCE Requirement: None
Cut-Off time since graduation: No limits set
Program offers couple match: Yes
Visas Sponsored or accepted: No visa

Texas Tech University Health Sciences Center Paul L Foster School of Medicine Emergency Medicine Residency Program

Specialty: Emergency Medicine
Program name: Texas Tech University Health Sciences Center Paul L Foster School of Medicine Program
Program code: 110-48-12-070

NRMP Code: 1710110C0
Program type: Community-based university affiliated hospital
State: Texas
Address: Texas Tech University HSC El Paso
4801 Alberta Ave, El Paso, TX 79905
Phone: (915) 545-7333
Fax: (915) 545-7338
Percentage of IMGs in the program: 0%
Minimum USMLE Step 1 Score Requirement: 210
Minimum USMLE Step 2 Score Requirement: 210
Attempts on any step: Must pass on first attempt
CS required at time of application: Yes including ECFMG certificate
USCE Requirement: Yes, 1 month
Cut-Off time since graduation: No limits set
Program offers couple match: Yes
Visas Sponsored or accepted: J1 visa

University of Texas School of Medicine at San Antonio Emergency Medicine Residency Program

Specialty: Emergency Medicine
Program name: University of Texas School of Medicine at San Antonio Program

Program code: 110-48-00-214
State: Texas
Address: University of Texas School of Medicine San Antonio
       7703 Floyd Curl Dr, San Antonio, TX 78229-3900
Phone: (210) 567-1183
Fax: (210) 567-0757
Percentage of IMGs in the program: 0%
Minimum USMLE Step 1 Score Requirement: No limits set
Minimum USMLE Step 2 Score Requirement: No limits set
Attempts on any step: No limits set
CS required at time of application: No
USCE Requirement: None
Cut-Off time since graduation: No limits set
Program offers couple match: Yes
Visas Sponsored or accepted: J1 visa

University of Texas Southwestern Medical School (Austin) Emergency Medicine Residency Program

Specialty: Emergency Medicine
Program name: University of Texas Southwestern Medical School (Austin) Program
Program code: 110-48-00-211
State: Texas

Address: University of Texas Southwestern Medical School Austin
              1400 IH 35 North, Austin, TX 78701
Phone: (512) 324-8221
Fax: (512) 324-8223
Percentage of IMGs in the program: 15%
Minimum USMLE Step 1 Score Requirement: No limits set
Minimum USMLE Step 2 Score Requirement: No limits set
Attempts on any step: No limits set
CS required at time of application: No
USCE Requirement: None
Cut-Off time since graduation: No limits set
Program offers couple match: Yes
Visas Sponsored or accepted: J1 visa

Utah

University of Utah Emergency Medicine Residency Program

Specialty: Emergency Medicine
Program name: University of Utah Program
Program code: 110-49-21-178
State: Utah

Address: University of Utah Medical Center
　　　　　30 N 1900 E, Salt Lake City, UT 84132
Phone: (801) 581-2272
Fax: (801) 585-0603
Percentage of IMGs in the program: 0%
(occasionally one)
Minimum USMLE Step 1 Score Requirement:
No limits set
Minimum USMLE Step 2 Score Requirement:
No limits set
Attempts on any step: No limits set
CS required at time of application: Yes
including ECFMG certificate
USCE Requirement: None
Cut-Off time since graduation: No limits set
Program offers couple match: Yes
Visas Sponsored or accepted: J1 visa

Virginia

Virginia Commonwealth University Health System Emergency Medicine Residency Program

Specialty: Emergency Medicine
Program name: Virginia Commonwealth University Health System Program

Program code: 110-51-21-160
NRMP Code: 1743110C0
Program type: University-based
State: Virginia
Address: Virginia Commonwealth University
Health System
          1250 E Marshall St, Richmond, VA
23298
Phone: (804) 828-4860
Fax: (804) 828-4603
Percentage of IMGs in the program: 0%
(occasionally one)
Minimum USMLE Step 1 Score Requirement:
No limits set
Minimum USMLE Step 2 Score Requirement:
No limits set
Attempts on any step: No limits set
CS required at time of application: No
USCE Requirement: Yes
Cut-Off time since graduation: No limits set
Program offers couple match: Yes
Visas Sponsored or accepted: J1 visa

University of Virginia Emergency Medicine Residency Program

Specialty: Emergency Medicine
Program name: University of Virginia Program
Program code: 110-51-21-125
State: Virginia

Address: University of Virginia Health System 1215 Lee St, Charlottesville, VA 22908-0699
Phone: (434) 982-1800
Fax: (434) 982-4118
Percentage of IMGs in the program: 0%
Minimum USMLE Step 1 Score Requirement: No limits set
Minimum USMLE Step 2 Score Requirement: No limits set
Attempts on any step: No limits set
CS required at time of application: No
USCE Requirement: None
Cut-Off time since graduation: No limits set
Program offers couple match: Yes
Visas Sponsored or accepted: J1 visa

Carilion Clinic-Virginia Tech Carilion School of Medicine Emergency Medicine Residency Program

Specialty: Emergency Medicine
Program name: Carilion Clinic-Virginia Tech Carilion School of Medicine Program
Program code: 110-51-13-209
NRMP Code: 1748110C0
Program type: Community-based university affiliated hospital
State: Virginia

Address: Carilion Clinic
1906 Belleview Ave, Roanoke, VA 24014
Phone: (540) 853-0182
Fax: (540) 981-9550
Percentage of IMGs in the program: 0%
Minimum USMLE Step 1 Score Requirement: No limits set
Minimum USMLE Step 2 Score Requirement: No limits set
Attempts on any step: No limits set
CS required at time of application: Yes including ECFMG certificate
USCE Requirement: Yes 6 months in the U.S., Canadian, or British systems
Cut-Off time since graduation: 5 years
Program offers couple match: Yes
Visas Sponsored or accepted: J1 visa

Eastern Virginia Medical School Emergency Medicine Residency Program

Specialty: Emergency Medicine
Program name: Eastern Virginia Medical School Program
Program code: 110-51-12-050
NRMP Code: 2980110C0
Program type: Community-based university

affiliated hospital
State: Virginia
Address: Eastern Virginia Medical School
        600 Gresham Dr, Norfolk, VA 23507
Phone: (757) 388-3397
Fax: (757) 388-2885
Percentage of IMGs in the program: 0%
Minimum USMLE Step 1 Score Requirement:
No limits set
Minimum USMLE Step 2 Score Requirement:
No limits set
Attempts on any step: Must pass on first
attempt including CS exam
CS required at time of application: No
USCE Requirement: None
Cut-Off time since graduation: No limits set
Program offers couple match: Yes
Visas Sponsored or accepted: J1 visa

Washington

University of Washington Emergency Medicine Residency Program

Specialty: Emergency Medicine

Program name: University of Washington Program
Program code: 110-54-31-210
State: Washington
Address: Harborview Medical Center
          325 Ninth Ave, Seattle, WA 98104
Phone: (206) 744-8334
Fax: (206) 744-4097
Percentage of IMGs in the program: 0%
Minimum USMLE Step 1 Score Requirement: 220
Minimum USMLE Step 2 Score Requirement: 220
Attempts on any step: Must pass on first attempt
CS required at time of application: No
USCE Requirement: Yes including one SLOE
Cut-Off time since graduation: No limits set
Program offers couple match: Yes
Visas Sponsored or accepted: J1 visa and H1b visa on select basis

West Virginia

West Virginia University Emergency Medicine Residency Program

Specialty: Emergency Medicine
Program name: West Virginia University Program
Program code: 110-55-21-128
NRMP Code: 1837110C0
Program type: University-based
State: West Virginia
Address: West Virginia University HSC
　　　　　One Medical Center Dr, Morgantown, WV 26506-9149
Phone: (304) 293-7215
Fax: (304) 293-6702
Percentage of IMGs in the program: 0%
Minimum USMLE Step 1 Score Requirement: No limits set
Minimum USMLE Step 2 Score Requirement: No limits set
Attempts on any step: No limits set
CS required at time of application: Yes including ECFMG certificate
USCE Requirement: Yes
Cut-Off time since graduation: 5 years
Program offers couple match: Yes
Visas Sponsored or accepted: J1 visa

Wisconsin

University of Wisconsin Emergency Medicine Residency Program

Specialty: Emergency Medicine
Program name: University of Wisconsin Program
Program code: 110-56-13-184
NRMP Code: 1779110C0
Program type: University-based
State: Wisconsin
Address: University of Wisconsin Hospitals and Clinics
          600 Highland Ave, Madison, WI 53792
Phone: (608) 890-8682
Fax: (608) 265-8241
Percentage of IMGs in the program: 0%
Minimum USMLE Step 1 Score Requirement: 220
Minimum USMLE Step 2 Score Requirement: 220
Attempts on any step: Must pass on first attempt
CS required at time of application: No
USCE Requirement: None
Cut-Off time since graduation: No limits set
Program offers couple match: Yes
Visas Sponsored or accepted: J1 visa

Specialty: Emergency Medicine
Program name: Medical College of Wisconsin
Affiliated Hospitals Program
Program code: 110-56-12-052
State: Wisconsin
Address: Medical College of Wisconsin
9200 W Wisconsin Ave, Milwaukee,
WI 53226
Phone: (414) 805-6455
Fax: (414) 805-6464
Percentage of IMGs in the program: 0%
Minimum USMLE Step 1 Score Requirement:
No limits set
Minimum USMLE Step 2 Score Requirement:
No limits set
Attempts on any step: No limits set
CS required at time of application: No
USCE Requirement: None
Cut-Off time since graduation: 3 years
Program offers couple match: Yes
Visas Sponsored or accepted: J1 visa and H1b
visa

I wish you good luck.

Thank you for buying our book.

Please, Please and Please take a minute to review our book on Amazon.

**Match A Doc
Residency Guide**

www.matchadoc.com